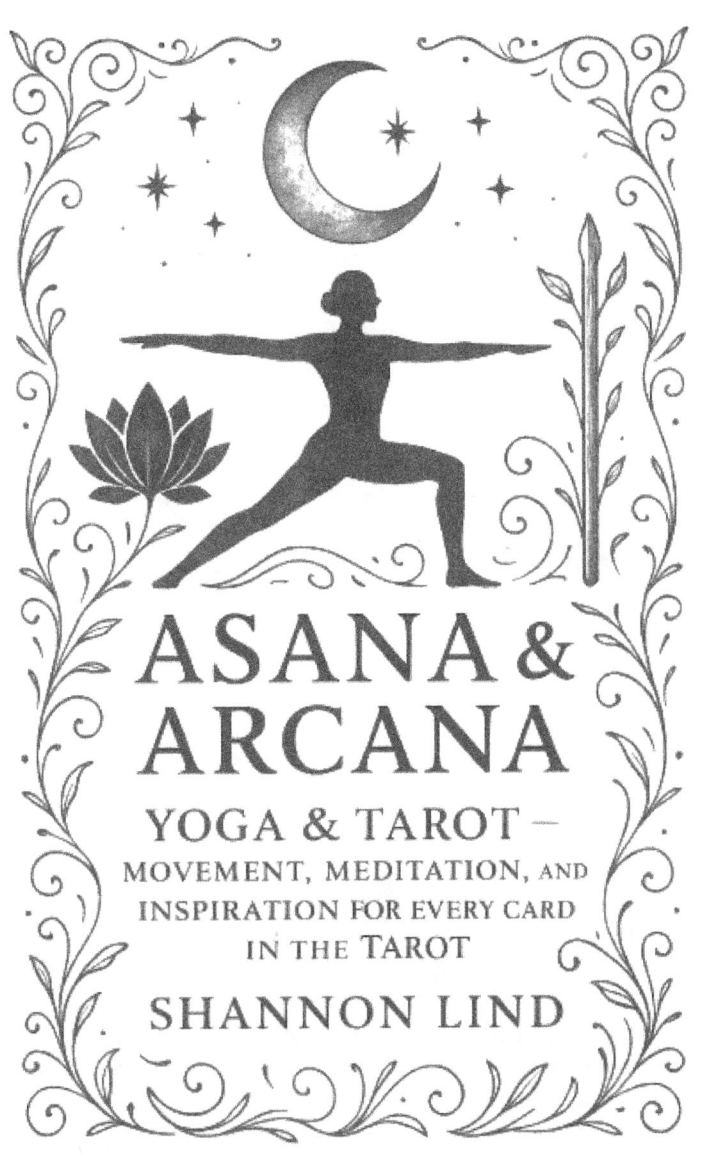

Published by 4Whiskers Publishing

Copyright © 2026 by 4Whiskers Publishing

All rights reserved. You may neither reproduce nor transmit any part of the contents of this book in any form or by any means, without the written permission of the publisher.

Although the publisher and the author have tried to ensure that the information in this book was correct at press time and while this publication provides accurate information regarding the subject covered, the publisher and the author assume no responsibility for errors, inaccuracies, omissions, or any other inconsistencies and disclaim any liability to any party for any loss, damage, or disruption caused by errors or omissions, whether such errors or omissions result from negligence, accident, or any other cause.

Printed and bound in the United States of America

First Printing

The information in this book is intended for general informational and educational purposes only. It is not a substitute for professional medical advice, diagnosis, or treatment. Always seek the advice of your physician or other qualified health provider before starting any new exercise program or making changes to your diet. Participation in any exercise program carries inherent risks, and you agree to participate at your own risk, holding the author and publisher harmless from any liability for injury or loss.

TABLE OF CONTENTS

THE MAJOR ARCANA — The Journey of the Soul	3
ASANAS AND WHY THEY WERE CHOSEN	3
CARDS AND CLASSES	7
THE REALM OF CUPS — Emotion, Intuition, Connection	37
ASANAS AND WHY THEY WERE CHOSEN	37
MUDRAS	39
PRANAYAMA	40
CARDS AND CLASSES	41
THE REALM OF WANDS — Fire, Inspiration, Action	57
ASANAS AND WHY THEY WERE CHOSEN	57
MUDRAS	60
PRANAYAMA	60
CARDS AND CLASSES	61
THE REALM OF SWORDS — Mind, Truth, Clarity	77
ASANAS AND WHY THEY WERE CHOSEN	77
MUDRAS	80
PRANAYAMA	80
CARDS AND CLASSES	81
THE REALM OF PENTACLES — Body, Earth, Stability	97
ASANAS AND WHY THEY WERE CHOSEN	97
MUDRAS	100
PRANAYAMA	100
CARDS AND CLASSES	101
COMPANION MATERIALS	117
TAROT SPREADS FOR YOGA	117
CLASS SHEET	139
USING THIS GUIDE FOR YOUR PRACTICE	147
CLOSING BLESSING	161
GLOSSARY	163

May this practice be a doorway.
A doorway into breath, into presence, into the quiet knowing that lives beneath thought.
As you step into this space, may the wisdom of your body rise to meet you.
May the archetypes of the tarot serve not as predictions but as gentle mirrors—guiding, clarifying, and revealing.

May the shapes you take remind you of your strength,
the breath you follow remind you of your softness,
and may the pauses between each movement remind you of the spaciousness available within you.

May your practice today be grounded in compassion,
guided by curiosity,
and held in the steady rhythm of your own becoming.

May every inhale draw you closer to yourself.
May every exhale set you free.

Blessed be this practice,
Blessed be this moment,
Blessed be the path that unfolds beneath your feet.

Shannon Lind
November, 2025

INTRODUCTION

As a yoga teacher with 15 years of experience, I sometimes struggle when it comes to choosing class themes. I would use the same three or four in rotation and, honestly, got tired of hearing myself; they grew to be just words empty of feeling and meaning.

At the same time, I was able to journal almost daily filling pages with thoughts, hopes, and words of self-encouragement. How was I able to find inspiration for personal uplifting thoughts, but run dry when it came to finding words to share with my students? The answer was simple: I was using beautiful tarot cards to inspire personal reflection and journaling.

Asana and Arcana was created as a meeting place between two profound inner traditions: the embodied wisdom of yoga and the archetypal language of the tarot. Each path has its own way of guiding us toward clarity, wholeness, and presence—tarot through symbolic insight, and yoga through breath, movement, and lived experience. When woven together, they form a powerful practice of reflection, sensation, and mindful inquiry.

Tarot offers us a symbolic mirror. Every card carries a universal theme—beginnings, intuition, courage, balance, disruption, transformation, joy, rest, and renewal. These are the same themes that arise on the yoga mat. As we breathe, move, strengthen, soften, and listen, we encounter the same archetypal moments the tarot teaches. The cards reflect the inner landscape; yoga offers the embodied path through it.

The themes in this book were developed by studying each card's core meaning, emotional tone, and psychological pattern, then translating those insights into the language of the body. What would The Fool feel like in movement? What breath belongs to The High Priestess? What posture expresses the balance of Justice or the surrender of The Hanged Man? I explored each card somatically and symbolically until the asanas, mudras, breathwork, and different limbs of yoga matched the card's energetic essence.

Every section begins with an introduction that includes thoughtfully chosen asanas, mudras, and pranayama practices. These were selected not only for their physical qualities, but for their emotional, spiritual, and symbolic resonance with each suit or arcana. The Major Arcana speaks to the soul's evolution; the four suits represent emotional, mental, creative, and physical life. Each has its own energy, its own rhythm, and its own way of being felt in the body.

This book is meant to meet you where you are—teacher, practitioner, seeker, or student. Whether you approach tarot symbolically, spiritually, or purely as storytelling, and whether your yoga practice is contemplative or dynamic, the integration of these two modalities opens a deeper, richer way of knowing yourself.

DEFINITIONS FOR THIS BOOK

Arcana
Tarot is a symbolic system of seventy-eight cards used for reflection, self-inquiry, and intuitive understanding. Rather than predicting the future, the tarot functions as a mirror—revealing inner patterns, emotional landscapes, and archetypal themes that shape the human experience. Every tarot deck is divided into the **Major Arcana**, which represent universal life lessons and spiritual milestones, and the **Minor Arcana**, which explore the day-to-day expressions of emotion, thought, action, and embodiment. In this book, tarot serves as a contemplative framework that supports yoga practice, offering imagery and metaphor that deepen awareness, intention, and personal insight.

Asana
Asana refers to the physical postures of yoga. While often understood simply as "poses," asana is more accurately a practice of alignment, stability, ease, and attentive presence within the body. The purpose of asana is not performance but embodiment—creating space, releasing tension, strengthening support, and cultivating mindful awareness. In this guide, asanas are chosen for their energetic resonance with each arcana group, helping practitioners explore tarot themes through movement and somatic experience.

Mudra
Mudra means "gesture" or "seal." These are symbolic hand positions—or sometimes full-body shapes—that redirect energy, focus the mind, and evoke specific emotional or spiritual states. Mudras can calm, energize, ground, or clarify depending on the gesture and intention. In this book, mudras are matched with each arcana group to amplify the qualities of the card—such as grounding for Pentacles,

inspiration for Wands, intuition for Cups, and clarity for Swords.

Pranayama

Pranayama refers to the intentional regulation of breath. The word combines *prana* (life force, energy, breath) and *ayama* (extension, expansion, or control). Through various techniques—such as Ujjayi, Nadi Shodhana, Kapalabhati, or deep diaphragmatic breathing—pranayama steadies the mind, balances the nervous system, and shifts the inner experience of practice. In this book, pranayama is curated for each arcana group to support the emotional and energetic themes of the cards.

Yoga

Yoga is a holistic system of physical, mental, energetic, and spiritual practices designed to cultivate awareness, presence, and union between body, breath, mind, and the deeper self. Rooted in ancient Eastern Indian philosophy, yoga is both a state of being (integration, wholeness) and a set of practices that help us remember that state. In this book, yoga is approached as an embodied path of self-inquiry—one that uses movement, breath, and mindfulness to illuminate inner wisdom, emotional clarity, and transformative growth.

The Eight Limbs of Yoga

The Eight Limbs of Yoga, described in Patanjali's *Yoga Sutra*, form a complete path toward self-awareness, ethical living, and spiritual integration. They are not linear steps but intertwined, mutually supportive practices.

Yama – Ethical foundations; how we relate to the world (non-harm, truthfulness, non-stealing, moderation, non-grasping).

Niyama – Inner observances; how we relate to ourselves (cleanliness, contentment, discipline, self-study, surrender).

Asana – Physical postures that prepare the body and mind for steady awareness.

Pranayama – Breath regulation that steadies, expands, and refines the flow of life force.

Pratyahara – Withdrawal from the senses; turning inward, away from external distraction.

Dharana – Focused concentration on a single point or intention.

Dhyana – Meditation; sustained, effortless awareness.

Samadhi – Integration; a sense of unity, peace, and connection with all things.

In this book, the Eight Limbs serve as a philosophical backbone. Each tarot card reflects aspects of these limbs—such as discipline (The Chariot), surrender (The Hanged Man), or integration (The World)—and the practices offered help guide practitioners toward deeper inner alignment.

HOW TO USE THIS BOOK

This compendium can be used in many different ways. It is both a reference and a companion to your favorite deck of tarot cards, meant to be explored intuitively. There is no "right" way—only the way that supports your practice, teaching, and inner inquiry.

1. As a Class-Planning Guide
The description of each tarot card includes:
- A Class Theme
- A Dharma Talk
- A Sankalpa or intention

It's worth noting that some cards are the embodiment of a mudra, or one of the eight limbs of yoga – it could be a yama, a niyama, asana, pranayama, pratyahara, dharana, dhyana, or samadhi. As these matches come up, we'll talk about the meaning of each.

You can use a single card to shape a full class, choose one card per week for a themed series, or explore the cards seasonally. Teachers may draw a card before class and use the corresponding themes to frame sequencing, language, and energetic focus.

2. As a Personal Practice Companion
Choose a card to guide your solo practice.
Let the Dharma Talk serve as reflection, then explore the recommended asanas, mudras, and breathwork. Allow the Sankalpa (Intention) to help you integrate the card's message in both mind and body.

3. As a Tarot Study Tool

The somatic interpretations help deepen the meaning of each card.
Movement and breath anchor the symbols in lived experience, offering insights that go beyond traditional card definitions.

4. As an Emotional or Spiritual Resource

When navigating transition, growth, or inner work, choose a card whose theme resonates and allow the embodied practices to support your process. This fusion of movement and metaphor can help soften fear, clarify intention, and cultivate resilience.

5. As a Creative Exploration

Feel free to adapt the material. Pair multiple cards, overlay suit energies, or use the meditations in journaling or ritual. The book is a springboard, not a prescription. I hope that you'll use the margins, blank pages, and other white space for your observations and explorations.

An Opening Note

Tarot shows us the story.
Yoga allows us to feel it.

Together they invite us into a life lived with awareness, presence, courage, and compassion.

This book is an offering for all who seek to walk their path with breath as guide and embodiment as truth.

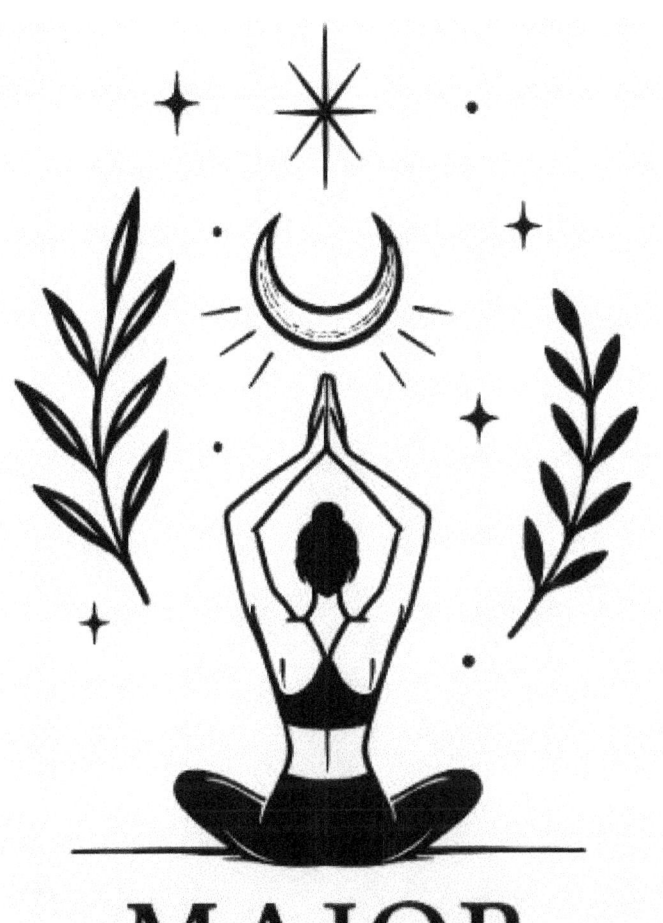

MAJOR ARCANA

THE MAJOR ARCANA — The Journey of the Soul

The Major Arcana represent the universal archetypes we encounter on the journey toward wholeness. The chosen asanas, mudras, and pranayama reflect grounding, readiness, intuitive listening, self-belief, and integration — each supporting the practitioner as they explore profound inner landscapes.

ASANAS AND WHY THEY WERE CHOSEN

Mountain Pose (Tadasana)
Represents presence, stability, and readiness.

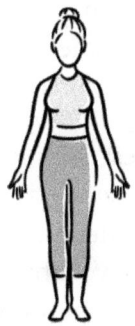

Cues: Stand with feet grounded hip width apart; arms down by your sides; palms facing forward.

Thoughts: Press evenly through the feet; lengthen the spine; soften the jaw; broaden the collarbones; let energy rise from the feet to the crown of your head.

MAJOR ARCANA

High Lunge (Ashta Chandrasana)
Symbolizes courageous forward movement and conscious choice.

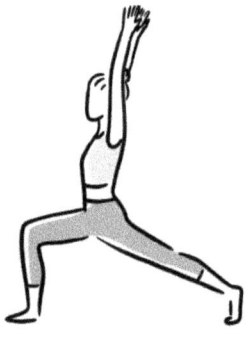

Cues: Start standing; step your foot forward and bend your front knee; keeping you back leg long and straight, come up onto the ball of your back foot; reach your arms high.

Thoughts: Stack front knee over ankle; reach through fingertips; draw ribs inward; soften shoulders.

Warrior I (Virabhadrasana I)
Embodies agency, self-belief, and intentional direction.

Cues: Start standing; step your foot forward and bend your front knee; keeping your back leg long and straight, keep your back heel on the ground; relax your hips toward the front of your mat; reach your arms high.

Thoughts: Press back heel down; lift chest without flaring ribs; root down as you rise.

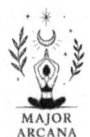

Tree Pose (Vrksasana)
Balances steadiness with adaptability and inner focus.

Cues: Start standing; shift your weight to one foot as rotate your other knee to the side while sliding that foot to the ankle or inner thigh of your standing leg; join hands together at heart center.

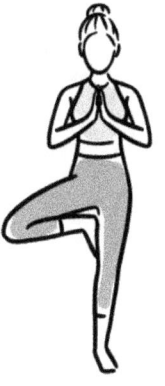

Thoughts: Press foot into inner leg; lengthen upward; steady the gaze; engage the core gently.

Seated Meditation
Supports inner clarity, introspection, and integration.

Cues: Take a comfortable seat; usually with ankles crossed and hands resting on thighs or knees.

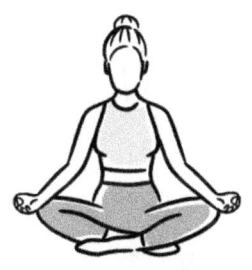

Thoughts: Sit tall; draw shoulders down; soften belly; deepen breath naturally.

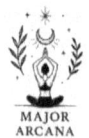

MUDRAS AND WHY THEY WERE CHOSEN

Gyan Mudra (Gesture of Insight)

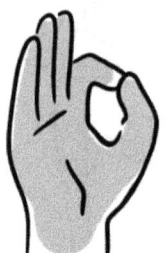

Encourages intuitive clarity, concentration, and inner guidance.

Touch the tip of your index finger to the tip of your thumb creating a circle. Keep other fingers relaxed.

Anjali Mudra (Gesture of Unity)

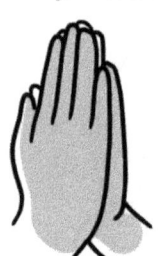

Aligns heart and mind, symbolizing devotion and integration. Also known as Prayer Hands.

Cues: Press your palms together nestling your thumbs into your chest to feel the vibration of your heart and the vibration of your breath.

PRANAYAMA AND WHY IT WAS CHOSEN

Ujjayi Breath (Ocean Breath)
Supports steadiness, presence, and deep awareness. Strengthens prana and grounds the mind.

Cues: Inhale through the nose; slight throat constriction; exhale as if fogging a mirror with lips closed; breath steady, audible, and grounding.

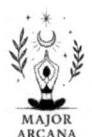

CARDS AND CLASSES

THE FOOL — Begin Again

Class Theme:
Stepping into the unknown with trust, presence, and breath.

Dharma Talk:
The Fool invites us to explore the sacred art of beginning — the moment where possibility expands before us and anything becomes possible. In yoga, this is felt each time we settle onto the mat and choose to meet the moment as it is, without past stories or future expectations. The Fool teaches the liberation that comes from openness and curiosity. When we allow ourselves to release anticipation and embrace spaciousness, we rediscover the joy of simply being.

This card shows us that readiness is not something we wait for; it is something we claim. Every inhale becomes an initiation, every exhale an invitation to trust. Through this lens, practice becomes a journey of exploration rather than accomplishment. The Fool asks: "What becomes possible when I step forward with wonder rather than fear?" The breath carries us toward that answer.

Sankalpa (Intention):
"I trust the step I cannot yet see."

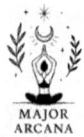

MAJOR ARCANA

THE MAGICIAN — You Already Have Everything You Need

Class Theme:
Awakening inner resources and stepping into creative power.

Dharma Talk:
The Magician reminds us that everything we need is already within us. This archetype teaches embodiment — the realization that your breath, awareness, intuition, and lived experiences form an inner toolkit that is always available. In yoga, this becomes the shift from performing poses to inhabiting them with intention and agency. The Magician invites us to gather our energy, attention, and purpose into a unified force.

This card also calls us to remember our inherent capability. Instead of searching outward, we turn inward with trust. The body becomes a vessel for creativity, the breath a tool for focus, and intuition a compass. When these aspects join, practice becomes an act of conscious creation. The Magician asks us: "Where can I trust my own power more deeply?" And the breath becomes our answer.

Sankalpa (Intention):
"Everything I need lives within me."

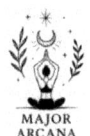

THE HIGH PRIESTESS — Trust the Quiet

Class Theme:
Deep listening, intuition, and the quiet spaces within.

Dharma Talk:
The High Priestess symbolizes intuition and the wisdom that arises when we soften our insistence on answers. This practice invites students into the subtle realm — sensation instead of performance, breath instead of analysis, feeling instead of striving. The High Priestess shows that the most profound truths arrive when the mind grows still enough to hear them. Through slow, intentional movement, we cultivate sensitivity to the body's quieter messages.

This archetype asks: "Where can I trust what I feel rather than what I think?" Yoga becomes a container for intuitive discovery, allowing layers of insight to reveal themselves without force. When we partner with our breath rather than control it, we step into a deeper form of knowing — one that is internal, ancient, and inherently wise.

Sankalpa (Intention):
"I trust the wisdom beneath the noise."

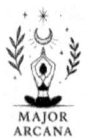

THE EMPRESS — The Art of Receiving

Class Theme:
Nourishment, softness, and embodied abundance.

Eight Limbs of Yoga:
Surrendering to the divine is the focus of both The High Priestess and the Niyama of Isvara Pranidhana. Intuition requires trusting yourself and the willingness to surrender to still the mind and accept the answers you're being given. Please consult the Hanged Man and the Ace of Wands for other ways to explore intuition.

Dharma Talk:
The Empress represents the sacred feminine principle of receptivity, creativity, and unconditional nurturing. This practice invites spaciousness in the body and gentleness in the breath. Instead of striving or pushing, we soften, open, and allow. The Empress teaches that receiving is not passive — it is active participation in the flow of life. Through conscious relaxation and self-honoring movement, we reconnect with our innate worthiness.

This archetype also speaks to the body as a vessel of abundance. When we approach movement with tenderness, we notice how the breath nourishes us from the inside out. The Empress asks: "What becomes possible when I soften instead of contract?" Through embodied receptivity, we cultivate a deep sense of belonging — not earned through effort, but recognized as already true.

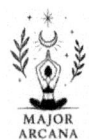

Sankalpa (Intention):
"I allow myself to receive."

Mudra:
In this case, the Adhara Mudra is a natural pairing with our Empress. Hands are held in front of heart or solar plexus. Press the little finger side of hands together, opening your thumbs to the other side (think about scooping water or cradling something precious).

Eight Limbs of Yoga:

In this case, The Empress is all that the Yama of Ahimsa is meant to be: non-harming, compassionate, and nurturing. You may also find these qualities in the Queen of Cups, Six of Cups, and the Four of Swords.

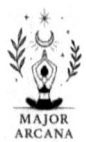
MAJOR ARCANA

THE EMPEROR — Root to Rise
Class Theme:

Structure, grounding, and steady self-leadership.

Dharma Talk:
The Emperor embodies stability, boundaries, and grounded authority. In practice, this becomes an exploration of structure — the alignment that keeps us steady, the breath that keeps us anchored, and the willpower that keeps us centered. The Emperor teaches that embodied strength arises not from rigidity but from clarity and intention. Each posture becomes an opportunity to root deeply and rise with purpose.

This archetype invites us to examine where we need stability in our lives. Through mindful alignment and conscious breath, we practice becoming unshakable while remaining compassionate. The Emperor asks: "How can I lead myself with strength and softness?" The mat becomes the place where we explore that balance.

Sankalpa (Intention):
"I rise from a grounded place."

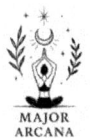

THE HEIROPHANT — The Wisdom in Practice

Class Theme:
Tradition, humility, and embodied wisdom.

Dharma Talk:
The Hierophant invites us to explore lineage — the teachings passed through time and breath. This archetype represents guidance, structure, and the rituals that shape our spiritual path.

He teaches that wisdom is lived, not memorized. Through steady practice, we embody what once was taught, transforming knowledge into experience.

Sankalpa (Intention):
Whisper: "I honor the wisdom that moves through me."

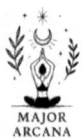

MAJOR ARCANA

THE LOVERS — Union Within

Class Theme:
Integration, harmony, and conscious connection.

Dharma Talk:
The Lovers represent the meeting place of choice and alignment. This archetype invites us to witness where our actions, beliefs, and desires meet.

It teaches that unity begins within. When breath, awareness, and intention align, we move from a place of wholeness rather than fragmentation.

Sankalpa (Intention):
Whisper: "I choose alignment with my truest self."

THE CHARIOT — Move with Intention

Class Theme:
Direction, discipline, and forward motion.

Dharma Talk:
The Chariot symbolizes self-directed momentum. Through clarity and willpower, we move intentionally toward growth.

This archetype teaches mastery over conflicting energies. With breath as a guide, we harness focus and inner strength.

Sankalpa (Intention):
Whisper: "My direction is chosen with clarity."

Eight Limbs of Yoga:
As does the Chariot, the Niyama of Tapas personifies discipline, effort, and moving ahead. Three other cards in the deck may also be read for this consideration: Eight of Pentacles, Seven of Wands, and Knight of Wands.

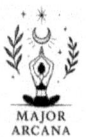

MAJOR ARCANA

STRENGTH — The Power of Softness

Class Theme:
Courage rooted in compassion, softness as strength.

Dharma Talk:
Strength teaches that true power is never forceful. Instead, it arises from deep inner steadiness, grounded presence, and emotional resilience. In yoga, this appears in the moments we meet challenge not with tension, but with breath. Strength calls us to soften where we grip, breathe where we resist, and expand where we contract. The symbology on the card of the lion represents our wild inner energies, and of the woman represents our capacity to meet them with tenderness.

This archetype asks us to redefine courage. It is not pushing past limits, but meeting ourselves with honesty and compassion. When we pair breath with awareness, we soften into what once felt overwhelming. Strength asks: "How can I be powerful without being hardened?" Through practice, we learn that gentleness is not the opposite of strength — it is the source of it.

Sankalpa (Intention):
"My softness is my strength."

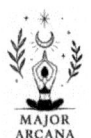

Eight Limbs of Yoga:

The Yama of Brahmacharya, or strength is well represented by the Strength card. It's strength with intention; passion with restraint; and using energy in the name of service. Other cards are the King of Wands and Two of Wands.

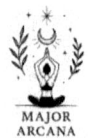

MAJOR ARCANA

THE HERMIT — Seek the Light Within

Class Theme:
Inner illumination, introspection, and sacred solitude.

Dharma Talk:
The Hermit symbolizes the quiet inner journey — the moments when we step away from noise and enter the sanctuary of our own wisdom. In yoga, this is the invitation to listen more deeply: to breath, to sensation, to intuition. Rather than seeking outward answers, we turn inward with curiosity and patience. The Hermit guides us toward the still places where truth reveals itself without being forced.

This archetype teaches that solitude is not loneliness but spacious clarity. When we turn down the volume of the world, we can finally hear our own voice. The Hermit asks: "What truth becomes audible when everything else becomes quiet?" Through mindful movement and intentional breath, we practice following that inner lantern — step by step, breath by breath.

Sankalpa (Intention):
"My inner light guides me."

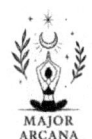

Eight Limbs of Yoga:

Few other cards and Niyamas are such a picture-perfect match as The Hermit and Svadhyaya. The Hermit is the epitome of introspection, introversion, and honoring self-knowledge. Svadhyaya is defined as self-study and inner work. More cards devoted to learning and inner contemplation are the Page of Pentacles, Two of Swords, and the Queen of Swords.

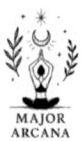

MAJOR ARCANA

WHEEL OF FORTUNE — Flow with Change

Class Theme:
Cycles, transition, and trusting the unfolding.

Dharma Talk:
The Wheel of Fortune reflects the cyclical nature of life — rise and fall, expansion and contraction, beginnings and endings. In yoga, we experience these cycles with every breath: the fullness of the inhale, the release of the exhale, and the pause in between. This card invites us to witness change without clinging or resistance. When we stop trying to fix ourselves at a single point, we rediscover the ease of flowing with life's natural rhythm.

This archetype teaches surrender to movement and acceptance of transformation. The Wheel does not ask us to control the cycle, but to partner with it. Through practice, we explore the interplay between steadiness and fluidity. The Wheel asks: "How can I trust the turning?" When we meet change with curiosity instead of fear, we align ourselves with the deeper currents of life.

Sankalpa (Intention):
"I trust the rhythm of my unfolding."

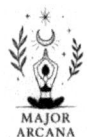

JUSTICE — Balance in All Things

Class Theme:
Truth, alignment, and clear self-reflection.

Dharma Talk:
Justice asks us to examine our inner alignment — to notice where our actions, thoughts, and values are in harmony and where they diverge. In yoga, this becomes a practice of honesty: observing where we over-effort, where we collapse, where we avoid, and where we lean in. Justice teaches that balance is not static; it is a dynamic, moment-to-moment recalibration guided by awareness.

This card also represents truth — not as a judgment, but as clarity. When we approach ourselves with compassion and transparency, we begin to see our patterns without shame or denial. Justice asks: "What truth am I ready to acknowledge?" Through breath and mindful movement, we learn to stand in integrity with ourselves.

Sankalpa (Intention):
"I stand in truth. I stand in balance."

Eight Limbs of Yoga:
Justice well represents the Yama of Satya or truthfulness, clear communication, and balanced action. This is also supported by the Ace of Swords and Page of Swords.

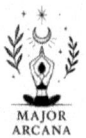
MAJOR ARCANA

THE HANGED MAN — Surrender and See Anew

Class Theme:
Perspective, surrender, and finding wisdom in stillness.

Dharma Talk:
The Hanged Man teaches the transformative power of surrender — not as defeat, but as spacious release. This archetype represents the moment we stop pushing against what is and instead soften into acceptance. In yoga, this is the pause that allows the body to integrate, the breath to deepen, and the mind to shift from striving to listening. The Hanged Man invites us to explore upside-down perspectives, both literally and symbolically.

This card reveals that clarity often comes when we stop insisting on our own timing and allow life to unfold. Through conscious surrender, we discover new layers of insight and possibility. The Hanged Man asks: "What changes when I let go?" Through breath-supported stillness, we allow wisdom to arise naturally.

Sankalpa (Intention):
"In surrender, I see more clearly."

Asana: Occasionally, a card speaks to a specific asana. Nowhere is this so clear as the Hanged Man with inversions. Inversions – when your head is below your heart level -- can have a calming influence and are known to improve focus due to the increased blood flow to the brain.

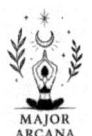

Eight Limbs of Yoga:

The Hanged Man is the perfect representation the Yama of Aparigraha or non-attachment. This, too, shall pass and we will be the better for it. We are able to release what no longer serves us in order to make room for what does. For continued guidance reflect on the Four of Cups and the Eight of Cups.

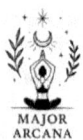

DEATH — The Gift of Letting Go

Class Theme:
Release, transformation, and surrendering what no longer serves.

Dharma Talk:
Death is not an ending — it is an alchemical turning point. This archetype guides us into the sacred act of releasing what has become too large, too heavy, or too untrue to carry forward. In yoga, this is the moment we soften into a forward fold, surrender into an exhale, or release tension we didn't realize we were holding. Death invites us to practice letting go not as loss, but as liberation. Every breath-out becomes a tiny initiation into spaciousness.

This card also reminds us that transformation requires trust. Just as the body renews itself breath by breath, we are constantly being invited into the next version of ourselves. When we release the familiar, even if it once protected us, we make room for new clarity and possibility. Death asks: "What am I ready to lay down so that I may rise lighter?" Through practice, we honor endings as sacred gateways.

Sankalpa (Intention):
"I release what no longer supports my becoming."

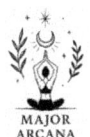

TEMPERANCE — The Middle Way

Class Theme:
Harmony, moderation, and the alchemy of balanced effort.

Dharma Talk:
Temperance invites us into the art of blending — effort with ease, discipline with softness, aspiration with surrender. In yoga, this is the steady middle path between pushing too hard and holding back too much. Temperance teaches that the wisest practices are those rooted in patience and presence. When we meet ourselves gently and consistently, we discover the alchemy of sustainable transformation.

This archetype also calls us into the energetic balance of opposites. The breath becomes the meeting place where fire and water coexist, where expansion and grounding take turns, where strength and tenderness merge. Temperance asks: "How can I cultivate harmony in my practice and my life?" Through mindful movement, we explore the spaces where balance emerges naturally, without force.

Sankalpa (Intention):
"I walk the path of harmony."

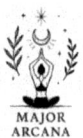

Asana:

Samasthiti is a combination of Tadasana (Mountain Pose) and Samasti Mudra. Mountain Pose is a grounded standing pose performed with both feet equally weighted and pressed into the earth. Samasti Mudra is made when both hands are pressed equally together with the thumbs nestled into the chest.

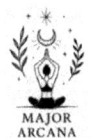

THE DEVIL — Liberation from Attachment

Class Theme:
Shadow work, truth-telling, and breaking unconscious patterns.

Dharma Talk:
The Devil represents the illusions that keep us small — the habits, fears, and narratives that pull us away from our inner truth. In yoga, this is the moment we become aware of gripping, bracing, or disconnecting from breath. The Devil invites radical honesty: not to shame the self, but to liberate it. When we see clearly the chains we have forged through old patterns, we regain the power to unmake them.

This archetype teaches that awareness is the first step toward freedom. When we shine a compassionate light on what binds us, we dissolve its power. The Devil asks: "What pattern am I ready to release?" Through breath and embodied presence, we move from unconscious reaction into conscious choice.

Sankalpa (Intention):
"I choose freedom over fear."

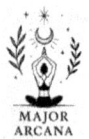
MAJOR ARCANA

THE TOWER — The Beauty of Breaking Open

Class Theme:
Sudden change, revelation, and the truth that emerges from disruption.

Dharma Talk:
The Tower represents the collapse of what is false, outdated, or unstable. Though its energy can feel shocking, it is ultimately a clearing — making space for truth to rise. In yoga, this is the moment a posture reveals imbalance or misalignment we were avoiding. The Tower teaches that destruction is not punishment; it is revelation. When the old structure falls, clarity floods in.

This archetype encourages us to trust the wisdom of upheaval. What breaks apart was never meant to hold our becoming. The Tower asks: "What truth is breaking through?" Through grounding breath, we rebuild ourselves with greater authenticity.

Sankalpa (Intention):
"I rise from what has fallen away."

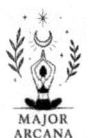

MAJOR ARCANA

THE STAR — Hope and Healing

Class Theme:
Replenishment, renewal, and the gentle return of trust.

Dharma Talk:
The Star arrives after disruption, offering healing, calm, and the slow return of hope. It invites us to tend to ourselves gently and to remember that healing is a process, not a performance. In yoga, this is the soft surrender of child's pose, the spacious breath after effort, or the subtle shimmer of calm after challenge. The Star teaches that hope is not naive — it is restorative.

This archetype invites us back into trust — trust in ourselves, in the path ahead, and in the light that persists even in uncertainty. The Star asks: "Where am I ready to soften and receive healing?" Through spacious breath, we let nourishment flow back in.

Sankalpa (Intention):
"I am held. I am healing."

Eight Limbs of Yoga:
The Star washes away heaviness and restores alignment which translates nicely to the guidance of the Niyama of Sauca or purity and cleanliness. It is the ideal of symbolic cleansing and spiritual clarity. Look to the Ace of Cups, Page of Cups, and Six of Swords for more direction.

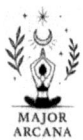

MAJOR ARCANA

THE MOON — Trust the Mystery

Class Theme:
Intuition, the subconscious, and navigating uncertainty with breath.

Dharma Talk:
The Moon represents what lies beneath the surface — dreams, intuition, shadow work, and the emotional tides that guide us. In yoga, this is the subtle shift in sensation, the instinctive movement, the quiet truth beneath thought. The Moon invites us to explore what is felt but not yet understood. It teaches that uncertainty is not a threat but a threshold.

This archetype illuminates illusions and fears — not to overwhelm us, but to free us from confusion. The Moon asks: "What truth lies beneath my fear?" Through slow, intuitive movement, we deepen trust in our inner knowing.

Sankalpa (Intention):
"I trust the mystery unfolding within me."

THE SUN — Joy in Motion

Class Theme:
Radiance, clarity, and moving from the heart with confidence.

Dharma Talk:
The Sun symbolizes vitality, joy, and embodied freedom. Its warmth encourages us to inhabit ourselves fully, without fear of shining. In yoga, The Sun is felt in expansive movement, in heart-openers, and in breath that feels bright and effortless. The Sun teaches that joy is medicine — a resource that reconnects us to our essence.

This archetype celebrates authenticity and the confidence that grows when we embrace who we truly are. The Sun asks: "Where am I ready to step into my full radiance?" Through uplifting breath and movement, we cultivate clarity and heart-centered joy.

Sankalpa (Intention):
"My light is welcome here."

Eight Limbs of Yoga:
Nothing brings more contentment than basking in the warmth of the sun. The Niyama of Santosa encourages acceptance of time spent in peacefulness and safety. Other warm cards include the Nine of Cups, Ten of Pentacles, and Four of Wands.

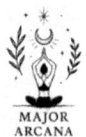

JUDGMENT — Awakening

Class Theme:
Revelation, inner calling, and rising into a higher version of self.

Dharma Talk:
Judgment symbolizes awakening — a call to rise into integrity, purpose, and transformation. In yoga, this is the moment we recognize our patterns and choose differently, not from shame but from clarity. Judgment invites deep reflection rooted in compassion, asking us to release outdated stories so we can live from truth.

This archetype opens a doorway into self-forgiveness and renewal. It invites us to listen inwardly for the voice that calls us toward our highest becoming. Judgment asks: "What truth is calling me forward?" Through mindful movement and introspective breath, we prepare to step into alignment.

Sankalpa (Intention):
"I awaken to myself."

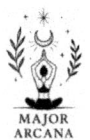

THE WORLD — Wholeness and Completion

Class Theme:
Integration, fulfillment, and arriving fully in oneself.

Dharma Talk:
The World represents the culmination of a journey — the moment where all lessons integrate into embodied wisdom. In yoga, this is savasana after meaningful practice, the place where everything lands. The World teaches that wholeness is a felt sense of belonging to oneself, cultivated over time and through devotion.

This archetype also signals new beginnings. Completion is not finality; it is readiness. The World asks: "What does it feel like to arrive?" Through breath and gentle awareness, we celebrate our journey while opening to what comes next.

Sankalpa (Intention):
"I am whole. I am complete."

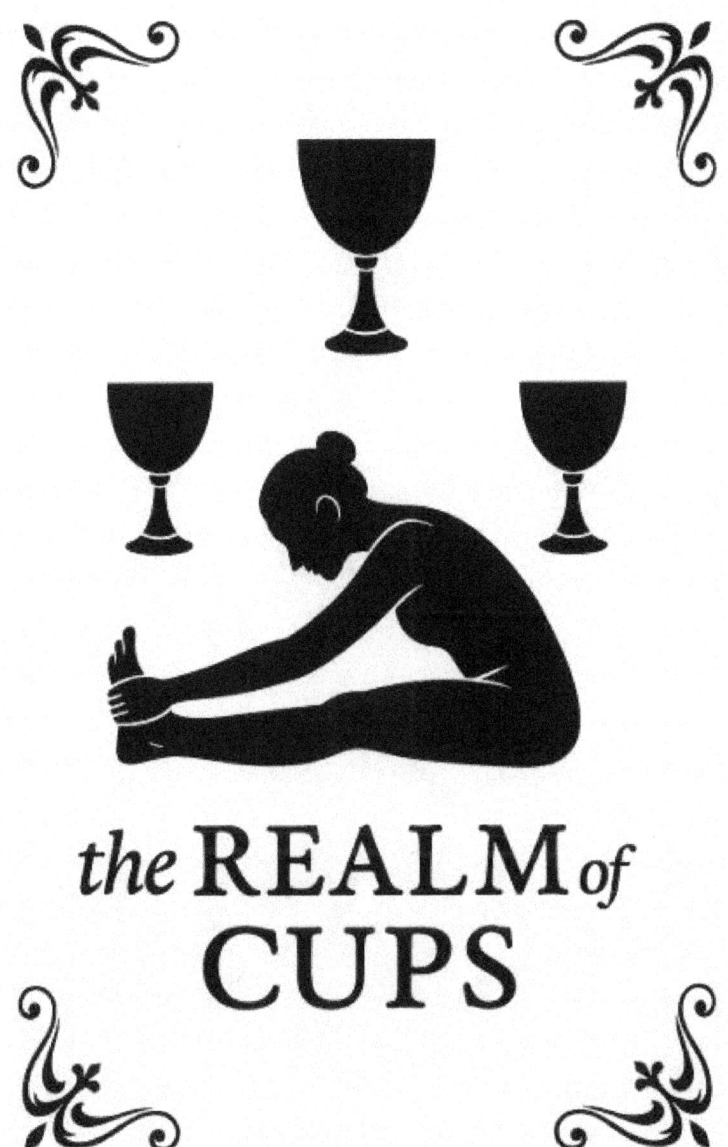

the REALM of CUPS

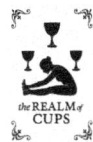

THE REALM OF CUPS — Emotion, Intuition, Connection

The Suit of Cups corresponds to the element of water, representing emotion, intuition, relationships, receptivity, and the inner tides of the heart. These practices emphasize fluidity, softness, emotional clarity, and gentle inward listening. Hatha yoga is a partner practice to the realm of Cups.

ASANAS AND WHY THEY WERE CHOSEN

Cat–Cow (Marjaryasana–Bitilasana)
Supports emotional fluidity and gentle heart-opening.

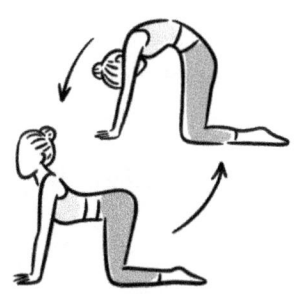

Cues: Start on hands and knees; on an exhale drop your chin to your chest; press into your hands to widen your shoulder blades; press your back to the sky. On an inhale lift your chin to look forward; press your chest forward; and lengthen your front body.

Thoughts: Move slowly with breath; soften shoulders; allow the spine to ripple. Appreciate the articulation of the spine.

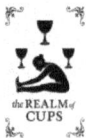

Seated Forward Fold (Paschimottanasana)
Invites emotional introspection and surrender.

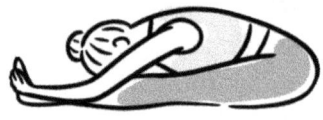

Cues: Start seated; gently drop your chest toward your thighs; hold your bellybutton to your spine; reach forward.

Thoughts: Lengthen spine first; fold from hips; release jaw; don't hesitate to use a strap held in each hand and around your feet to help you ease into the pose.

Low Lunge (Anjaneyasana)
Creates open, receptive space in the front body.

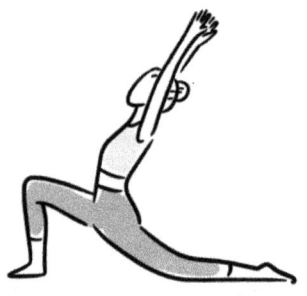

Cues: Start standing; step your foot forward and bend your front knee; lower your back knee to the Earth; reach your arms high.

Thoughts: Relax gently; lift heart; sink into hips.

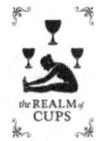

Reclined Bound Angle (Supta Baddha Konasana)
Encourages vulnerability, rest, and heart-softening.

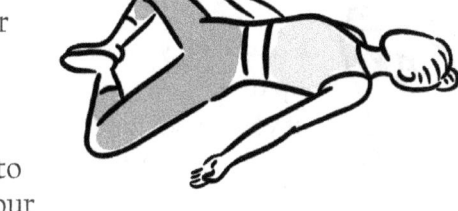

Cues: Lie on your back; bring the soles of your feet together letting your knees open to the sides; relax your arms where they're comfortable.

Thoughts: Support thighs with blocks; soften belly; deepen breath.

MUDRAS

Varuna Mudra — Gesture of Water

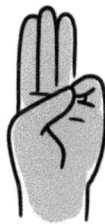

Enhances emotional flow and inner cleansing.

Cues: Touch the tip of your little finger to the tip of your thumb. The other fingers remain extended and relaxed.

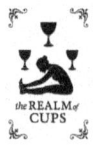

Hridaya Mudra — Gesture of the Heart

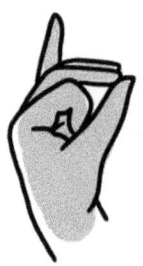

Supports emotional openness and compassion.

Cues: Curl your index finger in to touch the tip to the base of your thumb. Touch the tips of your middle and ring fingers to the tip of your thumb. Your little finger remains straight and relaxed.

PRANAYAMA

Nadi Shodhana — Alternate Nostril Breath
Balances emotional states and increases clarity.

Cues: Gently close your right nostril with your thumb and inhale through the left, then close the left nostril with your ring finger of the same hand and exhale through the right. Continue by inhaling through the right, switching, and exhaling through the left. Think about taking slow, even breaths; softening your shoulders; and breathing as if the breath moves through the heart.

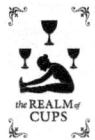

CARDS AND CLASSES

ACE OF CUPS — Opening to Emotion

Class Theme:
Receptivity, new emotional beginnings, and softening into the heart.

Dharma Talk:
The Ace of Cups symbolizes an overflowing well of emotional possibility — a fresh beginning, an invitation to feel more deeply, and a return to the heart's truth. It asks us to soften into receptivity rather than effort, to listen inwardly rather than push forward, to trust the quiet waters that rise within us. When we breathe into the chest, the heart responds — not with force, but with a widening, like ripples moving outward from a single drop. This card reminds us that emotional renewal does not come from striving, but from allowing: allowing ourselves to feel, to rest, to expand without agenda. In this moment, we sit at the edge of a full cup, witnessing what spills over when we stop containing ourselves. The Ace of Cups arrives when life is ready to move through us — when tenderness becomes strength, when vulnerability becomes a doorway, when love returns in its simplest, most unguarded form. Here, we practice opening gently, letting breath be the vessel and presence be the water. Here, we remember that the heart is not something to be earned, but something to be received.

Sankalpa (Intention):
"My heart opens with ease."

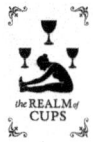

TWO OF CUPS — Connection and Harmony

Class Theme:
Union, partnership, and mutual understanding.

Dharma Talk:
The Two of Cups celebrates connection — not only with others, but with ourselves. It represents emotional reciprocity, presence, and the beauty of meeting another with openness. This card reminds us that relationship begins at the inner altar — how we speak to ourselves, how we listen to our own needs, how we honor what is tender and true. When we show up with authenticity, connection becomes effortless rather than earned. The Two of Cups teaches that intimacy is not about losing ourselves to union, but about bringing a whole, breathing self to the meeting point. This is where harmony is born — when two hearts stand equal, witnessed, and willing to be seen..

Sankalpa (Intention):
"I connect from wholeness."

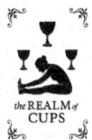

THREE OF CUPS — Joyful Community

Class Theme:
Celebration, friendship, and emotional uplift.

Dharma Talk:
The Three of Cups represents shared joy — the kind that lifts the spirit, nourishes the heart, and reminds us of the medicine of companionship. It invites us to remember what becomes possible when we gather, celebrate, and uplift one another. This card is a reminder that joy multiplies when shared — a single spark becoming a bonfire through presence and community. Here, we practice receiving support as fully as we offer it, letting ourselves be held in belonging. The Three of Cups asks us to honor our circles of care, to laugh often, to raise a glass or a heart in gratitude for the ones who walk with us.

Sankalpa (Intention):
"My joy is shared and multiplied."

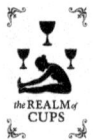

FOUR OF CUPS — Inner Reflection

Class Theme:
Turning inward, emotional clarity, and discernment.

Dharma Talk:
The Four of Cups asks us to pause, look inward, and become curious about our emotional landscape. It is a card of contemplation rather than withdrawal. This moment of stillness is not stagnation, but an invitation to notice where our attention rests, where we feel nourished, and where we feel numb. The Four reminds us that introspection is not a closing of the heart, but a clearing of space within it. When we sit with ourselves honestly, we may discover quiet blessings we once overlooked — offerings we were too busy, too guarded, or too tired to receive. This card invites us to turn toward our inner world with patience, letting insight surface like something remembered rather than learned..

Sankalpa (Intention):
"I listen to what my heart is truly asking."

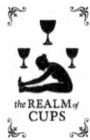

FIVE OF CUPS — Grief and Renewal

Class Theme:
Honoring loss, emotional release, and finding the path forward.

Dharma Talk:
The Five of Cups represents the tender process of grieving — acknowledging what has been lost while slowly turning toward what remains. This card teaches us that sorrow is not a failure of spirit, but a testament to what mattered. We are asked not to rush our healing, nor to minimize our pain, but to honor it with presence and breath. In time, awareness shifts: from the empty cups spilled before us to the ones still standing, full of possibility and life. The Five reminds us that healing is not about forgetting — it is about remembering ourselves again, piece by piece, in kindness.

Sankalpa (Intention):
"I honor my grief and my healing."

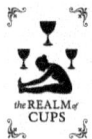

SIX OF CUPS — Memory and Innocence

Class Theme:
Nostalgia, sweetness, and returning to simplicity.

Dharma Talk:
The Six of Cups invites us to reconnect with innocence, memory, and the childlike qualities of joy and ease. It reminds us that there is wisdom in play, softness in simplicity, and healing in remembering who we were before the world asked us to harden. This card encourages us to approach life with curiosity rather than expectation, wonder rather than worry. When we return to what once delighted us — small joys, familiar comforts, old laughter — we touch a part of ourselves that is still whole, still bright, still unbroken. The Six of Cups teaches us that the past is not only a place of longing, but also a well of sweetness we can draw from in the present.

Sankalpa (Intention):
"I welcome simple, gentle joy."

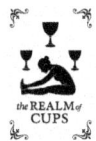

SEVEN OF CUPS — Clarity Amid Possibility

Class Theme:
Discernment, intuition, and choosing from truth.

Dharma Talk:
The Seven of Cups represents choices, dreams, and illusions. It invites clarity — the ability to sense which options nourish the heart. This card reminds us that not every desire is meant to be pursued, and not every glittering possibility is aligned with our wellbeing. When we feel pulled in many directions, the invitation is to pause, breathe, and listen for the quiet truth beneath the noise. The Seven asks us to choose not from urgency, fear, or fantasy, but from grounded intuition — the voice that rises only when we make space for it. Here we practice discernment, gently separating longing from illusion, vision from distraction, so we may step toward what is real and sustaining.

Sankalpa (Intention):
"I choose with clarity and intuition."

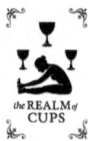

EIGHT OF CUPS — Walking Toward Truth

Class Theme:
Release, emotional courage, and choosing a higher path.

Dharma Talk:
The Eight of Cups symbolizes the brave moment when we turn away from what no longer nourishes us and move toward deeper authenticity. This card is not about rejection; it is about alignment. In yoga, this mirrors the moment we physically step out of a pose that is collapsing or forcing, and choose instead the shape that honors the body's truth letting your body shape the pose; not forcing your body to match the asana. The Eight teaches that emotional maturity requires discernment and self-listening.

This archetype asks us to trust the pull of the soul even when it leads us into the unknown. Growth often requires letting go — not in anger, but in clarity. The Eight asks: "What am I lovingly releasing so I can walk toward what is true?" Through breath and intentional movement, we practice stepping forward with courage and compassion.

Sankalpa (Intention):
"I walk toward what is true."

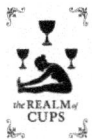

NINE OF CUPS — Emotional Fulfillment

Class Theme:
Contentment, gratitude, and savoring emotional abundance.

Dharma Talk:
The Nine of Cups is often called the "wish card," representing emotional satisfaction and heartfelt fulfillment. In yoga, this is the sensation after savasana when the breath feels spacious and the mind at ease. The Nine teaches us to pause and savor the goodness in our lives rather than racing toward the next goal. Gratitude becomes a practice, not a concept.

This archetype invites us to recognize the emotional abundance already present. Fulfillment is not something we chase; it is something we notice. The Nine asks: "Where can I savor what is already here?" Through gentle, appreciative movement, we settle into contentment.

Sankalpa (Intention):
"I savor the sweetness of this moment."

Asana:
Savasana or any other resting pose.

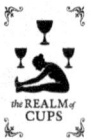

TEN OF CUPS — Emotional Harmony

Class Theme:
Wholeness, shared joy, and alignment between inner and outer worlds.

Dharma Talk:
The Ten of Cups symbolizes harmonious connection — the sense of emotional alignment within oneself and with community or chosen family. In yoga, this is embodied through heart-opening, balanced breath, and movement that feels integrated rather than fragmented. The Ten teaches that emotional harmony is found within first, then radiates outward.

This archetype invites us to celebrate connection and belonging. The Ten asks: "How can I cultivate inner harmony so that my outer world reflects it?" Through nourishing breath and mindful presence, we create a sense of emotional homecoming.

Sankalpa (Intention):
"Joy flows freely through me."

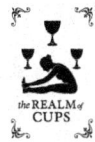

PAGE OF CUPS — Emotional Curiosity

Class Theme:
Openness, imagination, and intuitive exploration.

Dharma Talk:
The Page of Cups embodies childlike wonder, emotional playfulness, and intuitive curiosity. In yoga, this energy emerges when we approach movement without judgment — exploring novelty, softness, and imagination. The Page teaches that emotional wisdom can arrive in surprising, nonlinear ways.

This archetype encourages us to listen to the subtle nudges of intuition rather than dismissing them. The Page asks: "Where am I being invited to explore with a softer heart?" Through fluid, exploratory movement, we reconnect with emotional creativity.

Sankalpa (Intention):
"I explore with curiosity and openness."

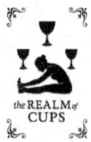

KNIGHT OF CUPS — Heart-Led Action

Class Theme:
Romanticism, inspiration, and moving from feeling.

Dharma Talk:
The Knight of Cups symbolizes following the heart's calling — pursuing dreams, creativity, or emotional truth with devotion. In yoga, this appears in the willingness to move with emotional honesty: stepping into a pose not out of ego, but out of intuitive knowing. The Knight teaches intentional, heart-led action.

This archetype invites us into motion guided by feeling rather than force. The Knight asks: "Where is my heart leading me?" Through breath and flowing transitions, we practice embodied inspiration.

Sankalpa (Intention):
"I move from the wisdom of my heart."

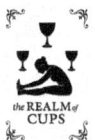

QUEEN OF CUPS — The Compassionate Heart

Class Theme:
Empathy, emotional depth, and inner calm.

Dharma Talk:
The Queen of Cups is the embodiment of emotional intelligence, compassion, and intuitive healing. In yoga, this is the practice of listening inwardly without judgment, responding with tenderness, and allowing emotions to be present without overwhelm. The Queen teaches emotional spaciousness — the ability to feel deeply while remaining grounded.

This archetype invites us to nurture ourselves and others with gentle awareness. The Queen asks: "How can I hold myself with more compassion?" Through soft breath and soothing movement, we cultivate inner calm.

Sankalpa (Intention):
"My heart is spacious and compassionate."

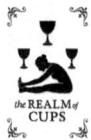

KING OF CUPS — Emotional Mastery

Class Theme:
Steadiness, emotional maturity, and balanced leadership.

Dharma Talk:
The King of Cups represents emotional stability — the ability to remain centered while experiencing deep feeling. In yoga, this is the balance between sensation and awareness, effort and ease. The King teaches that emotional mastery is not suppression, but integration.

This archetype invites us to lead from emotional wisdom: grounded, calm, and responsive. The King asks: "How can I remain anchored while the waters around me shift?" Through breath-supported movement, we cultivate steadiness of heart.

Sankalpa (Intention):
"My heart remains steady and clear."

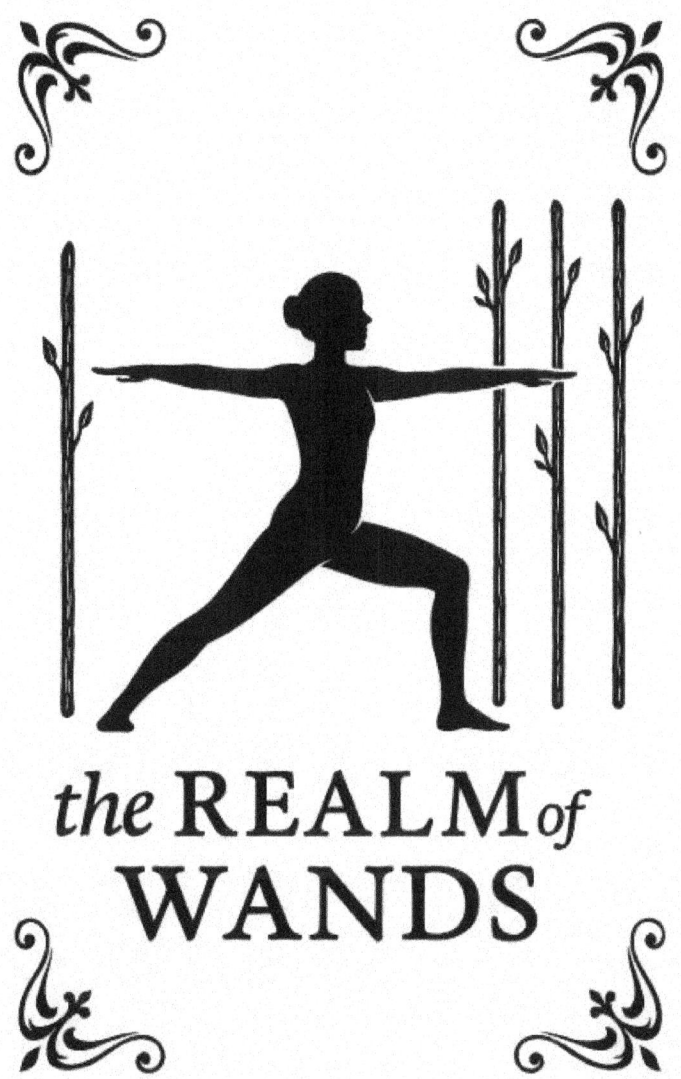

the REALM of WANDS

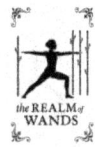

THE REALM OF WANDS — Fire, Inspiration, Action

The Suit of Wands corresponds to fire: creativity, passion, willpower, direction, and inspired movement. Practices in this suit emphasize heat-building, focus, intentional action, and aligned energy. A vinyasa practice is an ideal pairing to the realm of Wands.

ASANAS AND WHY THEY WERE CHOSEN

High Lunge (Ashta Chandrasana)
Ignites focus and strengthens direction.

Cues: Start standing; step your foot forward and bend your front knee; keeping you back leg long and straight, come up onto the ball of your back foot; reach your arms high.

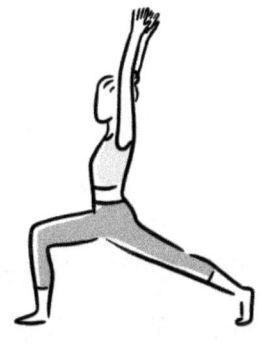

Thoughts: Press through back heel; lift chest; draw ribs inward; steady gaze.

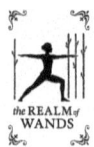

Warrior II (Virabhadrasana II)
Represents clarity of direction and sustained strength.

Cues: Start standing; step your foot forward and bend your front knee; spin your back foot so that the outside edge is roughly parallel to the back edge of your mat; front heel to back arch alignment; stretch your arms out from the shoulders; gaze over your front fingers.

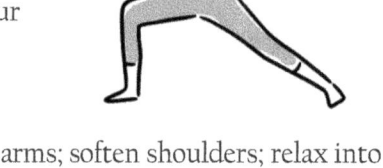

Thoughts: Press into outer edge of back foot; lengthen arms; soften shoulders; relax into hips.

Chair Pose (Utkatasana)
Builds heat, willpower, and grounded activation.

Cues: Stand tall, knees together; bend your knees as if sitting in a chair; shift your weight to your heels; reach your arms high.

Thoughts: Sit back; lengthen spine; engage core; lift heart.

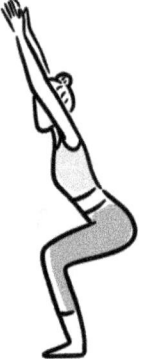

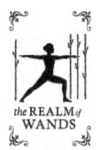

Goddess Pose (Utkata Konasana)
Emphasizes empowered presence and creative fire.

Cues: Step your feet wide apart; turn toes out about 45 degrees; bend your knees, sitting into your hips; keep your torso straight up and down – don't let yourself tilt forward; stretch your arms out from your shoulders and bend your elbows into a cactus shape.

Thoughts: Knees track over toes; tailbone heavy; chest lifted; strong and steady breath.

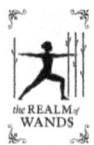

MUDRAS

Agni Mudra — Gesture of Fire

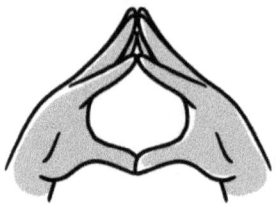

Supports activation, determination, and inner power.

Cues: Touch the tip of your ring finger to the base of your thumb. Allow your thumb to rest on top of your ring finger to apply gentle pressure. Your other fingers are straight and relaxed.

Hakini Mudra — Gesture of Mind and Focus
Enhances concentration, vision, and mental clarity.

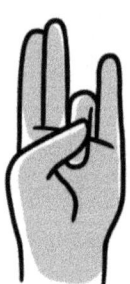

Cues: Touch the tips of the fingers of one hand to the tips of the corresponding fingers on the other hand pressing firmly. Palms face each other but are not touching. Keep your hands at heart level.

PRANAYAMA

Kapalabhati — Skull-Shining Breath
Builds heat, clears stagnation, and awakens willpower.

Cues: Passive inhale; sharp exhale; maintain steady rhythm; energize core.

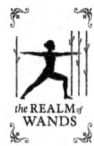

CARDS AND CLASSES

ACE OF WANDS — Spark of Inspiration

Class Theme:
New beginnings, creative ignition, and bold enthusiasm.

Dharma Talk:
The Ace of Wands is pure inspiration — the spark that lights the inner fire. It symbolizes a surge of energy, a new idea, or an intuitive impulse that wants expression. In yoga, this is the moment the body feels awake and ready, when breath moves freely, and creativity stirs in the chest. The Ace teaches us to trust the fire of possibility.

This archetype invites boldness and curiosity. Not every spark becomes a flame, but honoring inspiration is a sacred act. The Ace asks: "What wants to awaken within me?" Through energizing movement and intentional breath, we make space for new creative currents.

Sankalpa (Intention):
"I welcome the spark within."

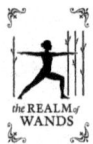

TWO OF WANDS — Vision and Possibility

Class Theme:
Planning, expanding perspective, and intentional direction.

Dharma Talk:
The Two of Wands represents the moment of vision — when we pause, survey our landscape, and consider what paths are available. In yoga, this is the breath before movement: the moment of choosing direction. The Two teaches that action becomes meaningful when it aligns with intention.

This archetype invites us to imagine with clarity and courage. The Two asks: "What direction feels true?" Through steady breath and grounding shapes, we explore the energy of choosing with purpose.

Sankalpa (Intention):
"My vision leads me with clarity."

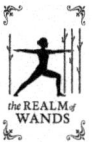

THREE OF WANDS — Expansion and Forward Momentum

Class Theme:
Progress, anticipation, and moving into broader horizons.

Dharma Talk:
The Three of Wands symbolizes growth in motion — the moment when we've chosen a direction and begin witnessing early signs of expansion. In yoga, this is the shift from intention to embodiment, where breath and action align. The Three teaches that progress unfolds with patience and openness.

This archetype invites us to hold space for what is emerging. The Three asks: "What is ready to expand?" Through energizing movement, we cultivate readiness and trust.

Sankalpa (Intention):
"I open to expanding possibilities."

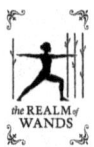

FOUR OF WANDS — Celebration and Stability

Class Theme:
Joy, community, and embodied gratitude.

Dharma Talk:
The Four of Wands represents joyful stability — a moment of celebration, belonging, and shared support. In yoga, this is the uplifting sensation after a well-balanced practice. The Four teaches that joy is strengthened through connection and mindful acknowledgment.

This archetype invites a pause to honor how far we've come. The Four asks: "What can I celebrate right now?" Through heart-opening movement and steady breath, we welcome joy as a grounding force.

Sankalpa (Intention):
"I celebrate the harmony in my life."

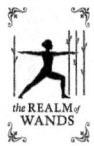

FIVE OF WANDS — Dynamic Energy

Class Theme:
Challenge, energetic friction, and constructive movement.

Dharma Talk:
The Five of Wands captures the energy of conflict — not as danger, but as dynamic motion. In yoga, this is the sensation of navigating challenge with breath and awareness. The Five teaches that friction can refine us when met with curiosity rather than resistance.

This archetype invites us to explore how we respond to intensity. The Five asks: "How can I stay centered amid chaos?" Through heat-building movement, we channel energy into productive focus.

Sankalpa (Intention):
"I stay centered as energy rises."

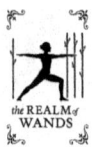

SIX OF WANDS — Recognition and Rising Confidence

Class Theme:
Achievement, visibility, and embodied self-trust.

Dharma Talk:
The Six of Wands symbolizes victory — not through ego, but through self-recognition and earned confidence. In yoga, this appears when we notice our own growth, strength, or resilience. The Six teaches us to honor our efforts without comparison.

This archetype invites us to stand tall and acknowledge our progress. The Six asks: "Where can I offer myself recognition?" Through expansive posture and empowering breath, we embody self-trust.

Sankalpa (Intention):
"I recognize my growth with gratitude."

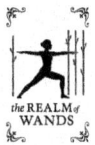

SEVEN OF WANDS — Holding Your Ground

Class Theme:
Boundaries, resilience, and steady determination.

Dharma Talk:
The Seven of Wands symbolizes standing firm in your truth despite challenge or external pressure. In yoga, this is the practice of maintaining alignment even when fatigue, doubt, or distraction appear. As B.K.S. Iyengar said, "The pose begins when you want to leave it." The Seven teaches that resilience grows from clarity and steady presence.

This archetype invites us to defend our energetic space with grounded confidence. The Seven asks: "Where am I ready to hold my ground?" Through strong, steady movement, we practice unwavering self-trust.

Sankalpa (Intention):
"I stand firmly in my truth."

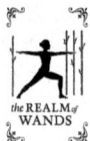

EIGHT OF WANDS — Swift Movement

Class Theme:
Momentum, clarity, and accelerated progress.

Dharma Talk:
The Eight of Wands represents rapid energy — the quickening of movement, ideas, and inspiration. In yoga, this is the sensation of flow when transitions feel effortless and breath guides motion without hesitation. This card teaches that sometimes life aligns swiftly, and our task is simply to keep pace with presence and clarity.

This archetype invites trust in momentum. When energy moves quickly, discernment becomes essential. The Eight asks: "How can I stay aligned even as I move swiftly?" Through breath-led sequencing, we practice clarity inside momentum.

Sankalpa (Intention):
"I move with clarity and purpose."

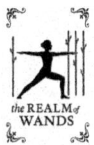

NINE OF WANDS — Resilience

Class Theme:
Endurance, boundaries, and wise perseverance.

Dharma Talk:
The Nine of Wands represents the moment of fatigue before a breakthrough — the last stretch of effort when weariness and determination coexist. In yoga, this appears in long holds, deep breaths, or the moment we choose not to collapse. The Nine teaches that resilience does not mean pushing past limits; it means staying present with what is.

This archetype invites wise perseverance. It asks: "How can I honor my effort while protecting my energy?" Through grounding breath and intentional pacing, we cultivate sustainable strength.

Sankalpa (Intention):
"My resilience is wise and grounded."

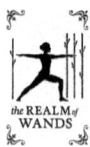

TEN OF WANDS — Release the Burden

Class Theme:
Overwork, responsibility, and laying down what is too heavy.

Dharma Talk:
The Ten of Wands symbolizes carrying too much — physically, emotionally, or energetically. In yoga, this is the tightness that accumulates when we clench, grip, or take on more than the body can hold. The concepts of sthira (steadiness and effort) and suka (ease, comfort) come to mind here: using strength and effort while at the same time leaning into softness and relaxation. The Ten teaches that burdens become lighter when they are acknowledged and released.

This archetype invites us to notice where we strain unnecessarily. The Ten asks: "What load am I ready to lay down?" Through releasing shapes and softening breath, we create space for relief.

Sankalpa (Intention):
"I release what is no longer mine to carry."

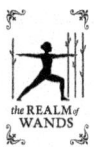

PAGE OF WANDS — Creative Beginnings

Class Theme:
Curiosity, exploration, and playful inspiration.

Dharma Talk:
The Page of Wands embodies youthful fire — adventurous, imaginative, and spirited. In yoga, this is the willingness to try new variations, explore unfamiliar shapes, or meet the practice with excitement instead of expectation. Yoga encourages us to explore and play with poses, movements, and sequences. The Page teaches that creativity thrives when we stay curious.

This archetype invites us to approach life with enthusiasm and openness. The Page asks: "Where am I ready to explore with fresh eyes?" Through free-flow movement, we awaken creative fire.

Sankalpa (Intention):
"I explore with joyful curiosity."

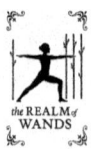

KNIGHT OF WANDS — Bold Action

Class Theme:
Passion, speed, and courageous movement.

Dharma Talk:
The Knight of Wands symbolizes daring action — the moment we leap toward what excites us. In yoga, this appears as the energetic transitions, the willingness to play, or the fiery breath that fuels motion. The Knight teaches passion balanced with intention.

This archetype invites boldness with awareness. The Knight asks: "Where is my passion asking me to move?" Through strong, direct sequencing, we embody courage.

Sankalpa (Intention):
"I move boldly and wisely."

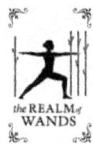

QUEEN OF WANDS — Radiant Confidence

Class Theme:
Magnetism, authenticity, and empowered presence.

Dharma Talk:
The Queen of Wands represents vibrant self-trust — the ability to shine without shrinking and to lead through authenticity. In yoga, this is the strength found in steady breath, lifted heart, and embodied alignment. The Queen teaches that confidence is not performance; it is presence.

This archetype invites us to embody our full expression. The Queen asks: "Where can I stand in my power with grace?" Through confident shapes and spacious breath, we honor our inner fire.

Sankalpa (Intention):
"My presence is powerful and authentic."

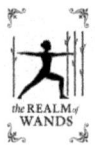

KING OF WANDS — Inspired Leadership

Class Theme:
Vision, mastery, and directing fire with wisdom.

Dharma Talk:
The King of Wands embodies mature fire — visionary, intentional, and steady in purpose. In yoga, this is the balance of heat and discipline, creativity and grounding. The King teaches us to direct our energy with clarity instead of impulse.

This archetype invites purposeful leadership of the self. The King asks: "How can I lead my life with inspired vision?" Through structured yet fiery sequences, we cultivate embodied empowerment.

Sankalpa (Intention):
"I lead with clarity, vision, and fire."

Pranayama:
Sitali Pranayama (Cooling Breath). Roll your tongue. Inhale your breath through the tongue as if you're sipping the air through a straw.

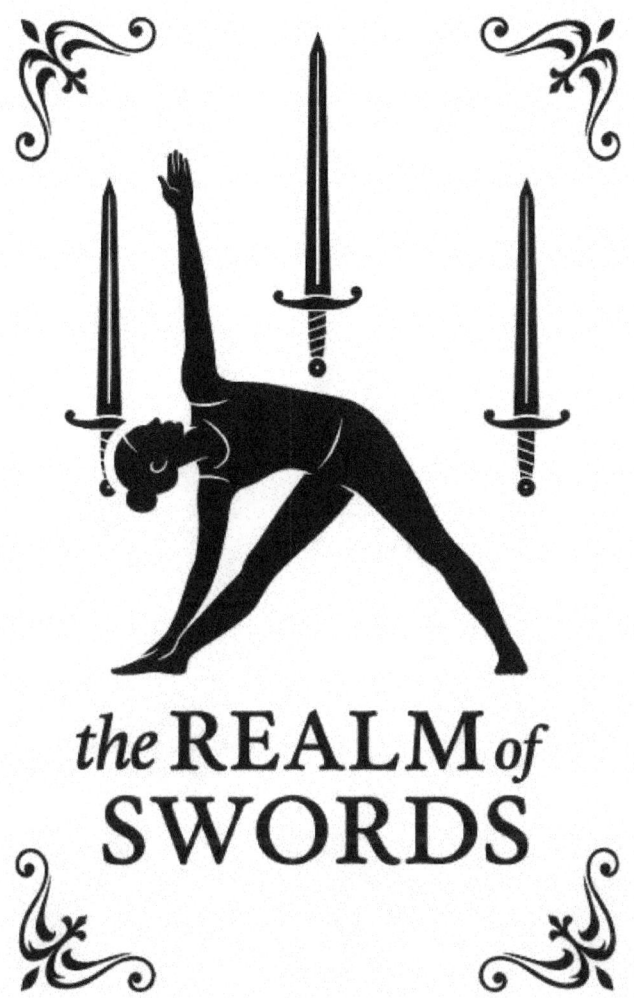

the REALM of SWORDS

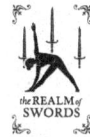

THE REALM OF SWORDS — Mind, Truth, Clarity

The Suit of Swords corresponds to the element of air, representing thought, communication, discernment, truth, and mental clarity. Practices in this suit emphasize sharp awareness, mental spaciousness, boundary-setting, and breath-led reflection.

ASANAS AND WHY THEY WERE CHOSEN

Standing Forward Fold (Uttanasana)
Calms the mind and lengthens the spine, offering mental quiet.

Cues: Start standing; hinge at your hips reaching your chest toward your thighs; let your neck hang long; option to connect your hands to the back of your calves to intensify the pose.

Thoughts: Release head; soften neck; bend knees as needed; breathe to the bottom of the lungs lengthening the back body.

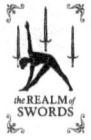

Triangle Pose (Trikonasana)
Invites clarity, expansion, and steady focus.

Cues: Start in Warrior 2 (see The Ream of Wands); straighten your front knee; reach your front arm forward to shift your ribs over your front leg; tilt your front arm down, reaching high with your back arm keeping your collar bones wide.

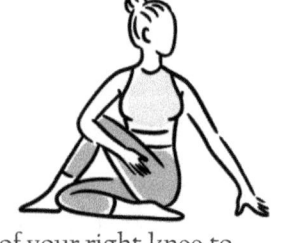

Thoughts: Root feet; lengthen side body; rotate rib cage; soften gaze.

Half Lord of the Fishes (Ardha Matsyendrasana)
Supports mental clarity and energetic release.

Cues: Start in seated meditation (see Major Arcana); cross your right leg over your left so the sole of your right foot is on the ground outside your left knee; twist to the right placing your right hand on the floor behind you; option to press your left elbow to the outside of your right knee to intensify the pose.

Thoughts: Ground sit bones; lengthen on inhale; twist gently on exhale.

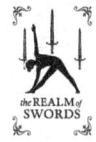

Plank Pose (Phalakasana)
Builds focus, discipline, and mental stamina.

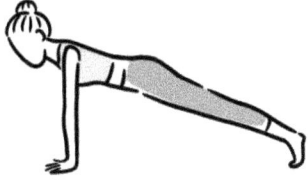

Cues: Start on all fours, knees under your hips and wrists in line with your shoulders; one at a time, step your feet out behind you to create a long line from your heels to the crown of your head.

Thoughts: Engage core; press floor away; lengthen heels back; steady breath.

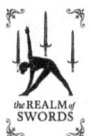

MUDRAS

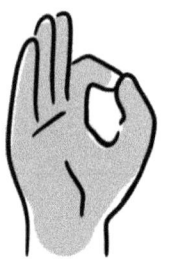

Hakini Mudra — Gesture of Mind and Focus
Supports concentration, memory, and mental integration.

Cues: Touch the tips of the fingers of one hand to the tips of the corresponding fingers on the other hand pressing firmly. Palms face each other but are not touching. Keep your hands at heart level.

Jnana Mudra — Gesture of Insight
Promotes clarity, wisdom, and inner truth.

Cues: Also known as Gyan Mudra (see the Major Arcana). Touch the tip of the index finger to the tip of the thumb creating a ring. Let the other fingers remain straight and relaxed.

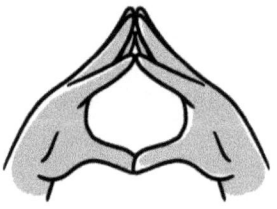

PRANAYAMA

Box Breath (Sama Vritti Variation)
Balances the nervous system and sharpens mental focus.

Cues: Inhale for four; hold for four; exhale for four; hold for four; maintain smooth breath cycles.

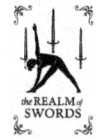

CARDS AND CLASSES

ACE OF SWORDS — Truth Awakens

Class Theme:
Mental clarity, breakthrough, and fresh insight.

Dharma Talk:
The Ace of Swords represents the sudden clarity that cuts through confusion — the moment truth arrives with precision. In yoga, this is the awareness that emerges when breath quiets the mind and reveals simplicity beneath complexity. The Ace teaches that truth is a liberation when it arises from inner clarity rather than force.

This archetype invites us to honor insight. The Ace asks: "What truth is becoming clear?" Through breath-led movement, we sharpen awareness and welcome mental spaciousness.

Sankalpa (Intention):
"I welcome the clarity I need."

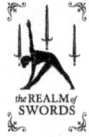

TWO OF SWORDS — The Pause Before Choice

Class Theme:
Stillness, indecision, and quiet inner listening.

Dharma Talk:
The Two of Swords symbolizes the crossroads — the moment where choice is required but clarity is not yet formed. In yoga, this is the pause between breaths, the brief stillness between movements. The Two teaches that decisions made from stillness rather than urgency hold greater truth.

This archetype invites us to listen inwardly. The Two asks: "What am I afraid to see?" Through gentle inward-focused practice, we soften into inner knowing.

Sankalpa (Intention):
"In stillness, clarity forms."

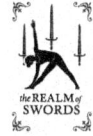

THREE OF SWORDS — Healing Through Truth

Class Theme:
Heartache, honesty, and emotional release.

Dharma Talk:
The Three of Swords represents the pain that comes from truth — the heartbreak, disappointment, or separation that pierces us. In yoga, this arises in the tender moments when we sit with discomfort rather than bypass it. The Three teaches that healing begins with acknowledgment.

This archetype invites us to feel fully and honestly. The Three asks: "What truth needs to be honored so I can heal?" Through breath-supported movement, we create space for emotional clarity.

Sankalpa (Intention):
"I allow truth to heal me."

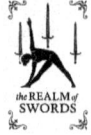

FOUR OF SWORDS — Rest the Mind

Class Theme:
Recovery, stillness, and restoring mental peace.

Dharma Talk:
The Four of Swords represents intentional rest — withdrawing from noise to restore clarity. In yoga, this is the embodied wisdom of savasana, child's pose, or any moment of surrender. The Four teaches that rest is not avoidance; it is integration.

This archetype invites deep restoration. The Four asks: "How can I honor my need for quiet?" Through gentle, supported shapes, we cultivate mental spaciousness.

Sankalpa (Intention):
"I rest into clarity."

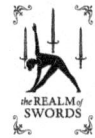

FIVE OF SWORDS — Honest Boundaries

Class Theme:
Conflict, self-protection, and the cost of misalignment.

Dharma Talk:
The Five of Swords symbolizes conflict — not always external, often internal. It reveals moments when we betray our own truth or act from ego rather than integrity. In yoga, this appears as pushing too hard, collapsing, or losing connection to breath. The Five teaches that boundaries clarify where our energy belongs.

This archetype invites honesty without self-judgment. The Five asks: "Where am I acting out of alignment?" Through mindful awareness, we reclaim clarity and integrity.

Sankalpa (Intention):
"I honor my truth with clarity and care."

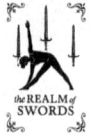

SIX OF SWORDS — Transition with Grace

Class Theme:
Moving on, mental relief, and crossing into calmer waters.

Dharma Talk:
The Six of Swords represents a necessary transition — leaving behind difficulty and moving toward peace. In yoga, this is the shift from agitation into calm, from strain into ease. The Six teaches that change does not require closure to be healing.

This archetype invites gentle forward motion. The Six asks: "What am I ready to move beyond?" Through smooth, flowing movement, we embody transition.

Sankalpa (Intention):
"I move toward peace."

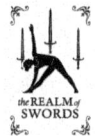

SEVEN OF SWORDS — Truth and Transparency

Class Theme:
Honesty, discernment, and revealing what is hidden.

Dharma Talk:
The Seven of Swords addresses avoidance, secrecy, or self-deception — the parts of ourselves we hide from. In yoga, this appears when we avoid sensations, skip breaths, or resist what arises. The Seven teaches compassionate self-honesty.

This archetype invites revelation without shame. The Seven asks: "What truth am I avoiding?" Through breath-led awareness, we practice transparency with ourselves.

Sankalpa (Intention):
"I meet my truth with compassion."

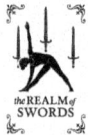

EIGHT OF SWORDS — Release from Limitation

Class Theme:
Mental boundaries, self-liberation, and inner clarity.

Dharma Talk:
The Eight of Swords depicts self-imposed limitation — the moments when fear, doubt, or habit keep us feeling stuck. In yoga, this is the experience of gripping, overthinking, or believing a shape is unavailable before we've even tried. The Eight teaches that many constraints dissolve when we soften into awareness rather than tighten into fear.

This archetype invites us to notice where we confine ourselves with old stories. The Eight asks: "What belief is ready to loosen its hold on me?" Through gentle breath and spacious movement, we create room for mental freedom.

Sankalpa (Intention):
"I release the stories that hold me back."

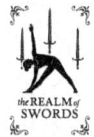

NINE OF SWORDS — Soften the Mind

Class Theme:
Anxiety, overthinking, and compassionate awareness.

Dharma Talk:
The Nine of Swords symbolizes mental overwhelm — sleepless worry, looping thoughts, and inner pressure. In yoga, this is the mind that won't quiet even when the body becomes still. Chitta Vritti, or Monkey Mind, is a yoga concept of the mind being constantly active and jumping around. The Nine teaches us to meet mental unrest with tenderness rather than judgment.

This archetype invites conscious compassion. The Nine asks: "How can I soothe my mind instead of fighting it?" Through slow, rhythmic breath and gentle inward-focused shapes, we practice softening spiraling thoughts.

Sankalpa (Intention):
"With compassion, my mind softens."

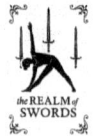

TEN OF SWORDS — The End of Mental Suffering

Class Theme:
Release, clarity after overwhelm, and conscious closure.

Dharma Talk:

The Ten of Swords represents the culmination of mental struggle — the moment we acknowledge something has reached its limit. In yoga, this is when we stop forcing, stop gripping, and surrender into a deeper truth. The Ten teaches that endings can be liberating when met with awareness.

This archetype invites radical acceptance. The Ten asks: "What am I ready to put down for good?" Through restorative shapes and grounding breath, we create space for renewal.

Sankalpa (Intention):
"I release the struggle and welcome peace."

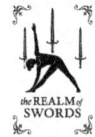

PAGE OF SWORDS — Curious Awareness

Class Theme:
New ideas, mental exploration, and thoughtful communication.

Dharma Talk:
The Page of Swords embodies intellectual curiosity — the desire to learn, clarify, and understand. In yoga, this is the part of us that loves alignment cues, seeks subtlety, and explores sensation with interest. The Page teaches the value of engaged, attentive presence.

This archetype invites open-minded discovery. The Page asks: "What new perspective is emerging?" Through alert but soft movement, we cultivate clarity and curiosity.

Sankalpa (Intention):

"I explore ideas with openness and clarity."

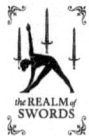

KNIGHT OF SWORDS — Focused Action

Class Theme:
Decisiveness, ambition, and mental precision.

Dharma Talk:
The Knight of Swords symbolizes direct, determined movement — the impulse to pursue truth or action quickly. In yoga, this energy appears in strong vinyasa, precise transitions, and moments of bold effort. The Knight teaches that clarity paired with discernment becomes powerful.

This archetype invites intentional action rather than scattered motion. The Knight asks: "Where is my focus leading me?" Through clear, purposeful sequences, we practice directing our energy with intelligence.

Sankalpa (Intention):
"My mind is clear, and my actions are aligned."

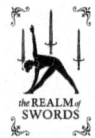

QUEEN OF SWORDS — Truth with Compassion

Class Theme:
Discernment, boundaries, and wisdom through clarity.

Dharma Talk:
The Queen of Swords embodies discerning truth — the ability to see clearly and speak honestly while remaining compassionate. In yoga, this is the practice of aligning with what is real rather than what is comfortable. The Queen teaches that clarity is a form of love.

This archetype invites us to honor our boundaries and insight. The Queen asks: "What truth am I ready to claim?" Through spacious breath and aligned movement, we cultivate honest awareness.

Sankalpa (Intention):
"My clarity is kind and true."

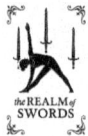

KING OF SWORDS — The Wisdom of the Mind

Class Theme:
Integrity, mental mastery, and thoughtful leadership.

Dharma Talk:
The King of Swords represents intellectual strength — not forceful, but principled and steady. In yoga, this is the clarity that arises when mind and breath align, when focus becomes spacious rather than tight. The King teaches leadership through wisdom rather than reaction.

This archetype invites clear thinking rooted in integrity. The King asks: "How can I lead my life with intelligence and fairness?" Through balanced, mindful movement, we cultivate mental mastery.

Sankalpa (Intention):
"I lead with clarity, wisdom, and integrity."

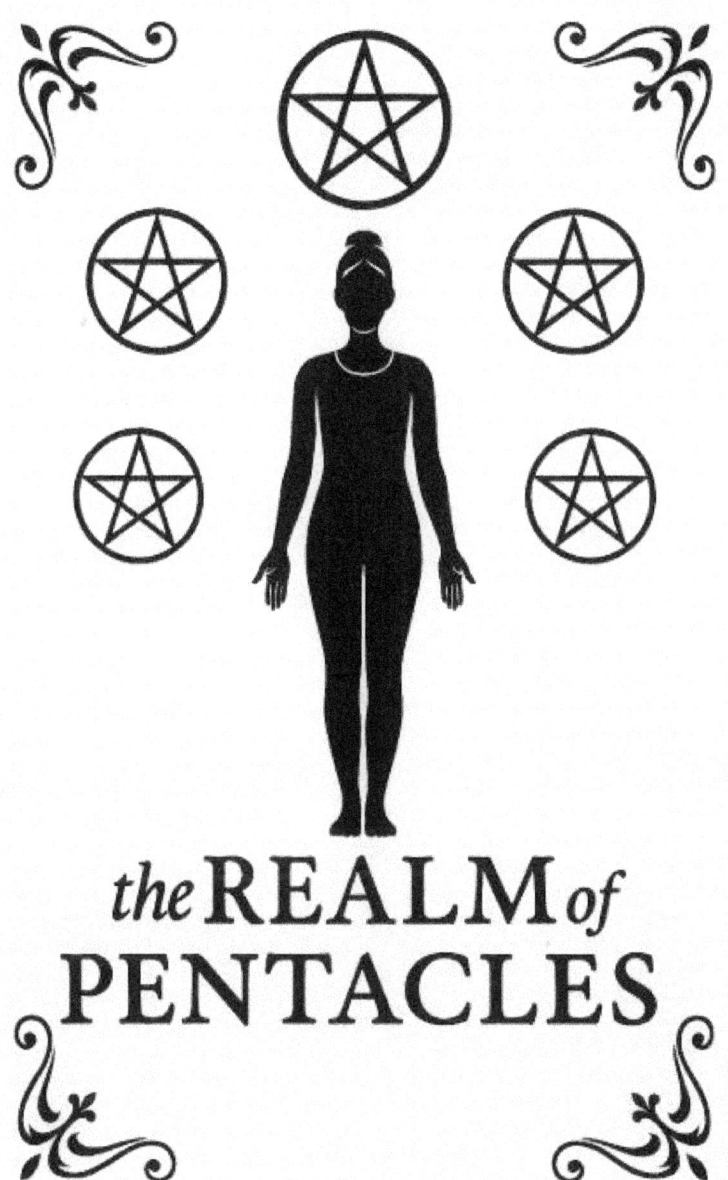

the REALM of PENTACLES

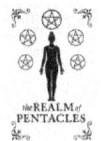

THE REALM OF PENTACLES — Body, Earth, Stability

Pentacles correspond to the element of earth: the physical body, grounding, material stability, daily life, work, and long-term growth. Practices in this suit emphasize steadiness, embodiment, patience, and grounded presence.

ASANAS AND WHY THEY WERE CHOSEN

Mountain Pose (Tadasana)

Represents foundation, embodiment, and grounded awareness.

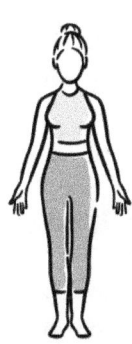

Cues: Stand with feet grounded hip width apart; arms down by your sides; palms facing forward.

Thoughts: Root through all four corners of the feet; lengthen upward; soften shoulders; breathe down into belly and legs.

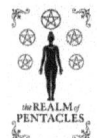

Tree Pose (Vrksasana)
Supports balance, rootedness, and inner steadiness.

Cues: Start standing; shift your weight to one foot as rotate your other knee to the side while sliding that foot to the ankle or inner thigh of your standing leg; join hands together at heart center.

Thoughts: Press standing foot down; engage core; lengthen upward; soften gaze.

Warrior I (Virabhadrasana I)
Builds strong foundations and aligned strength.

Cues: Cues: Start standing; step your foot forward and bend your front knee; keeping your back leg long and straight, keep your back heel on the ground; relax your hips toward the front of your mat; reach your arms high.

Thoughts: Anchor back heel; bend front knee; lift heart without flaring ribs.

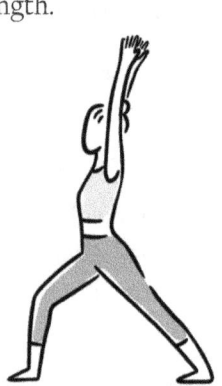

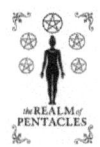

Bridge Pose (Setu Bandhasana)
Encourages slow-building strength and grounded expansion.

Cues: Lying flat, knees bent, soles of your feet on the ground; press into your feet to lift your hips and back; your weight should move to the top of your upper back; head and neck 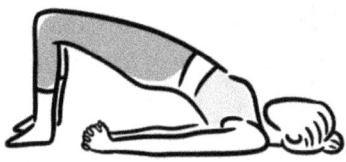 remain free and unweighted; option to clasp your hands underneath you to intensify the pose.

Thoughts: Press through feet; lift hips; draw shoulder blades together; breathe into chest.

Child's Pose (Balasana)
Invites grounding, rest, and connection to earth energy.

Cues: Kneel on the floor; open your knees; relax forward resting 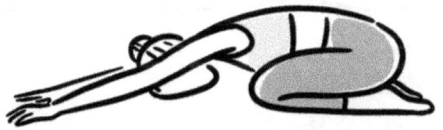 your torso on your thighs; your arms can be wherever they are the most comfortable, but they're generally stretched out in front of you.

Thoughts: Soften hips back; relax forehead; breathe into back body.

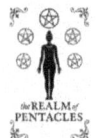

MUDRAS

Prithvi Mudra — Gesture of Earth

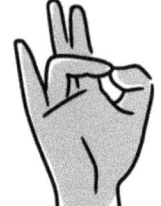

Encourages grounding, physical nourishment, and stability.

Cues: Touch the tip of the ring finger to the tip of the thumb. Other fingers remain straight and relaxed.

Bhumisparsha Mudra — Earth-Touching Gesture
Symbolizes rooted truth, stability, and connection with the earth.

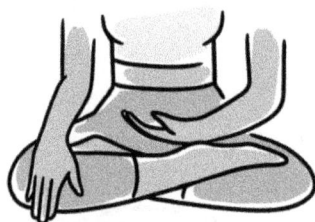

Cues: Sit comfortably with your left hand in your lap, palm facing up. Rest your right hand on your knee, palm facing down with fingers pointing toward the Earth.

PRANAYAMA

Sama Vritti — Equal Breath
Balances the nervous system and supports grounded presence.

Cues: Inhale for a count of four; exhale for a count of four; keep breath smooth and even.

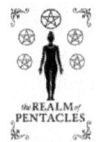

CARDS AND CLASSES

ACE OF PENTACLES — Planting the Seed

Class Theme:
New beginnings, grounding potential, and nurturing growth.

Dharma Talk:
The Ace of Pentacles represents a fresh start in the physical or material realm — a seed of possibility waiting to be planted. In yoga, this is the feeling of coming back into the body after distraction, rediscovering grounding and steady presence. The first yoga sutra (Yoga Sutra 1:1) teaches that yoga starts now: Atha Yoga Anushasanam. The Ace teaches that all long-term growth begins with a single intentional step and patient tending.

This archetype invites us to honor beginnings without rushing. Seeds take time, nourishment, and trust. The Ace asks: "What new intention am I ready to plant?" Through grounded movement and deep breath, we nurture sustainable growth from the ground up.

Sankalpa (Intention):
"I plant with intention."

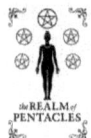

TWO OF PENTACLES — Balance in Motion

Class Theme:
Adaptability, flexibility, and steady presence amid change.

Dharma Talk:
The Two of Pentacles symbolizes the dance of balance — the shifting, flowing adjustments required to stay steady amid movement. In yoga, this is the subtle sway in Tree Pose or the rhythmic shift between transitions. Remember, the work is in the wobble. The Two teaches that balance is dynamic, not static.

This archetype encourages graceful adaptability. The Two asks: "Where am I being invited to rebalance?" Through gentle shifts and steady breath, we practice meeting change without losing center.

Sankalpa (Intention):
"I balance with grace."

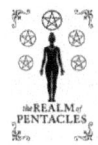

THREE OF PENTACLES — Co-Creation

Class Theme:
Teamwork, collaboration, and honoring each person's role.

Dharma Talk:
The Three of Pentacles symbolizes building together — progress created through collaboration, shared effort, and respect for each person's strength. In yoga, this appears in group energy, co-regulation, and learning through community. This could translate into practicing in a studio or with other bodies. The Three teaches that mastery grows through patience, integration, and cooperation.

This archetype invites us to acknowledge the value of shared creation. The Three asks: "Where can collaboration support my growth?" Through grounded practice, we recognize that we do not build alone.

Sankalpa (Intention):
"Together, we build with care."

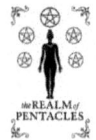

FOUR OF PENTACLES — Holding and Releasing

Class Theme:

Boundaries, control, stewardship, and softening the grip.

Dharma Talk:
The Four of Pentacles represents holding — sometimes necessary, sometimes constrictive. In yoga, this shows up as tension, rigidity, or bracing against sensation. The Four teaches discernment: when to protect energy and when to soften.

This archetype asks us to examine our relationship with control. The Four asks: "Where am I holding too tightly?" Through breath-supported release, we soften what no longer needs protection.

Sankalpa (Intention):
"I hold what matters and release the rest."

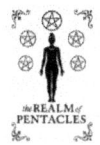

FIVE OF PENTACLES — Support and Belonging

Class Theme:
Hardship, resilience, and remembering we are not alone.

Dharma Talk:
The Five of Pentacles represents moments of difficulty — emotional, physical, or material. In yoga, this may arise as frustration with the body or a sense of disconnection. The Five teaches that even in hardship, support exists, often closer than we think.

This archetype invites us to seek connection and receive care. The Five asks: "Where can I let myself be supported?" Through grounding breath, we reconnect with belonging.

Sankalpa (Intention):
"Support surrounds me."

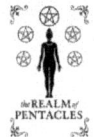

SIX OF PENTACLES — Giving and Receiving

Class Theme:
Generosity, reciprocity, and balanced exchange.

Dharma Talk:
The Six of Pentacles represents the natural rhythm of giving and receiving — inhalation and exhalation, effort and ease, offering and receiving. In yoga, this balance becomes a felt experience in breath and movement.

This archetype invites us to participate in the flow of generosity. The Six asks: "Where can I give freely? Where can I receive graciously?" Through balanced movement, we honor reciprocity.

Sankalpa (Intention):
"I give and receive in harmony."

Eight Limbs of Yoga:
The Six of Pentacles is the model of giving, fairness, and receiving. The Yama of Asteya teaches us not to take what isn't freely given and to have a generosity of spirit. Also look to the Nine of Pentacles for the same guidance.

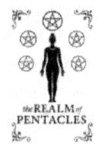

SEVEN OF PENTACLES — Patience and Assessment

Class Theme:
Reflection, long-term growth, and evaluating direction.

Dharma Talk:
The Seven of Pentacles symbolizes slow growth — progress that requires patience, tending, and honest reflection. In yoga, this is the gradual deepening over months or years, not moments. The Seven teaches us to pause, reflect, and adjust without self-judgment.

This archetype invites us to trust the process. The Seven asks: "What is growing, even if I cannot see it yet?" Through slow, intentional practice, we honor long-term cultivation.

Sankalpa (Intention):
"I trust in the time growth requires."

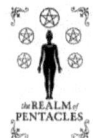

EIGHT OF PENTACLES — Devoted Practice

Class Theme:
Skill refinement, consistency, and loving the process.

Dharma Talk:
The Eight of Pentacles represents dedication — the steady, deliberate effort that strengthens skill and deepens awareness. In yoga, this is the repeated return to alignment, breath, and presence. The Eight teaches us that mastery is not an endpoint but a practice, cultivated moment by moment. When we show up consistently, even in small ways, transformation unfolds naturally.

This archetype invites us to honor the process rather than fixate on the outcome. The Eight asks: "What am I willing to devote myself to?" Through steady movement and mindful breath, we cultivate patience, discipline, and quiet pride in the work of becoming.

Sankalpa (Intention):
"I honor the practice that shapes me."

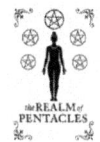

NINE OF PENTACLES — Self-Sufficiency and Ease

Class Theme:
Confidence, independence, and savoring the fruits of effort.

Dharma Talk:
The Nine of Pentacles symbolizes stability earned through consistent care and effort. In yoga, this is the spacious ease that arises after deep practice — when the breath feels wide, the heart soft, and the body grounded. The Nine teaches us to trust our own resourcefulness and to enjoy the abundance we have cultivated through effort and intention.

This archetype invites us to savor what we often overlook in the rush toward the next task. Anchor your thoughts in the present while remaining mindful. The Nine asks: "Where can I pause and appreciate what I've created?" Through slow, luxurious movement, we embody independence, gratitude, and ease.

Sankalpa (Intention):
"I savor the abundance within and around me."

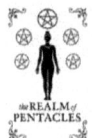

TEN OF PENTACLES — Legacy and Fulfillment

Class Theme:
Long-term security, community roots, and generational wellbeing.

Dharma Talk:
The Ten of Pentacles symbolizes lasting fulfillment — stability created through consistent choices, community support, and deep roots. In yoga, this is the sense of timelessness that arises when the body and breath rest in harmony. The Ten teaches us to honor the structures, relationships, and efforts that make long-term wellbeing possible.

This archetype invites reflection on the legacies we create — in our families, our communities, and our own bodies. The Ten asks: "What am I building that will endure?" Through grounding movement, we honor the foundations that support us and the ones we choose to pass forward.

Sankalpa (Intention):
"My roots are deep, and my life is supported."

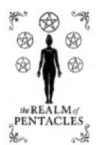

PAGE OF PENTACLES — Learning Through the Body

Class Theme:
Curiosity, grounded learning, and new possibilities.

Dharma Talk:
The Page of Pentacles represents a student's mindset — grounded curiosity, hands-on learning, and willingness to begin again. In yoga, this is the playful exploration of alignment, the gentle study of sensation, and the fresh perspective that arises when we treat every posture as new. The Page teaches us that learning is embodied.

This archetype invites us to make space for experimentation without judgment. The Page asks: "What new skill or awareness is ready to take root?" Through grounded breath and slow exploration, we cultivate humility and excitement for growth.

Sankalpa (Intention):
"I learn with patience and presence."

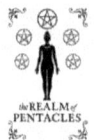

KNIGHT OF PENTACLES — Steady Devotion

Class Theme:
Consistency, responsibility, and grounded commitment.

Dharma Talk:
The Knight of Pentacles embodies dependable effort — slow, steady, thoughtful progress. In yoga, this is the practitioner who shows up even on the days when energy is low, choosing presence over perfection. The Knight teaches that commitment built on patience becomes unshakeable.

This archetype invites us to cultivate resilience through routine. The Knight asks: "Where can I commit with steadiness and care?" Through deliberate, rooted postures, we practice intentional effort supported by breath.

Sankalpa (Intention):
"My steps are steady and purposeful."

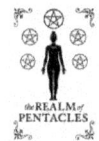

QUEEN OF PENTACLES — Nourishing Presence

Class Theme:
Care, comfort, and embodied generosity.

Dharma Talk:
The Queen of Pentacles embodies grounded compassion — nurturing the body, tending to the home, and cultivating wellbeing through practical care. In yoga, this is the practice of moving gently, honoring sensation, and choosing nourishment before ambition. The Queen teaches that care is a powerful form of strength.

This archetype invites us to tend to our needs with sincerity. The Queen asks: "How can I nourish myself more fully?" Through slow, restorative movement, we create a sanctuary within the body.

Sankalpa (Intention):
"I offer myself steady, loving care."

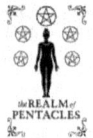

KING OF PENTACLES — Rooted Mastery

Class Theme:
Grounded leadership, abundance, and embodied stability.

Dharma Talk:
The King of Pentacles represents mature mastery — grounded, generous, dependable, and wise. In yoga, this is the deep confidence that arises after years of practice, when movement is steady and breath effortless. The King teaches that abundance grows from patience, integrity, and presence.

This archetype invites us to inhabit leadership rooted in service and steadiness. The King asks: "How can I lead my life from grounded wisdom?" Through strong, stable movement, we honor our connection to earth and the prosperity found in embodied presence.

Sankalpa (Intention):
"I lead with steadiness, wisdom, and ease."

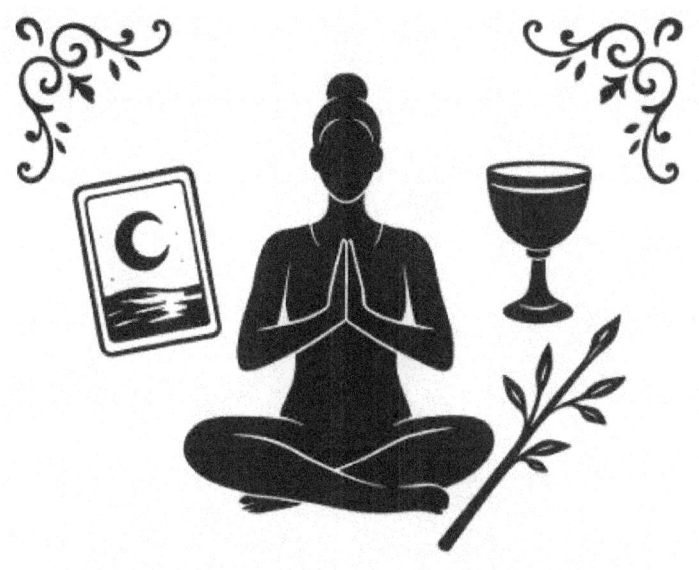

COMPANION MATERIALS

COMPANION MATERIALS

TAROT SPREADS FOR YOGA

Embodied tools for sequencing, intention-setting, and energetic alignment

These spreads were created to help teachers weave tarot wisdom into their classes with clarity and purpose or to help students open their creativity when exploring their home practice. Each spread invites reflection, creativity, and embodied movement. Use them before planning a class, when designing a series, or anytime you want inspiration from both symbolic and somatic sources.

Benefits of Using These Tarot Spreads

The tarot spreads in this book deepen the yoga journey by offering a reflective framework that helps practitioners clarify intention, understand emotional or energetic patterns, and align their practice with what is most needed in the moment. Each spread encourages mindful inquiry, guiding students and teachers toward insights that support sequencing, breathwork choices, and meaningful class themes. They help bridge inner awareness with embodied experience, transforming personal reflections into movement, meditation, and self-compassion. By revealing subtle layers of thought, emotion, and intuition, these spreads create a pathway for more intentional practice, richer teaching, and a fuller connection to the wisdom within.

These spreads are valuable because they offer a structured way to translate intuition into insight, helping practitioners understand what they are experiencing internally so they can meet it intentionally on the mat. Each spread highlights emotional, mental, or energetic themes that might otherwise remain beneath the surface; they allow the practitioner or teacher to shape movement, breath, and meditation around what is truly needed. By blending symbolic wisdom with embodied practice, the spreads turn yoga into a more personal, reflective, and meaningful experience. The cards encourage clarity, deepen self-awareness, and help practitioners connect the lessons of the tarot to their daily lives, creating a holistic practice that supports growth on every level — physical, emotional, and spiritual.

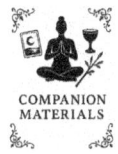

COMPANION MATERIALS

A teacher can use these tarot spreads privately as a planning tool, even if they prefer not to mention tarot during class. Each spread reveals an emotional, energetic, or thematic thread that can guide the tone of the practice, the sequencing, the pacing, the breathwork, and the dharma talk — without ever naming the card or the source of inspiration. Instead of telling students, "This class is based on the Seven of Cups," the teacher might simply offer the distilled theme: clarity, discernment, or mindful choice. The spreads help the teacher identify what qualities to emphasize: grounding vs. uplifting, softening vs. energizing Then direct the arc of the class in a way that feels cohesive and intentional. In this way, tarot becomes an invisible planning partner: a quiet, personal tool that enriches the teacher's creativity and insight while offering students a class experience rooted in meaningful, embodied themes they can connect to in their own way.

THE SEQUENCE BUILDER SPREAD

A spread for planning the flow, energy arc, and theme of a class.

Layout (three cards)

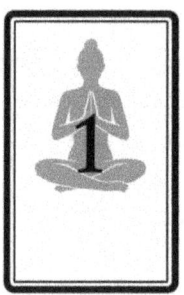 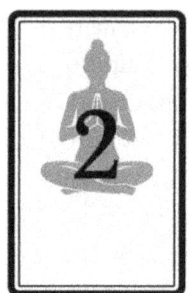 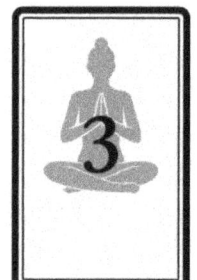

Card One — Opening Energy

What energy should open the class?
Use this card to determine the tone of the opening meditation, the first grounding shapes, or the breathwork that sets the container.

Card Two — Central Lesson

What is the heart of the class? What is the main teaching?
This card guides your Dharma Talk, signature pose, or central sequence.
Fire cards → stronger flows
Water cards → fluid mobility
Air cards → slow, mindful pacing
Earth cards → grounding and stability

Card Three — Closing Reflection

What needs to be softened, integrated, or reflected on?
Use this card to craft the Sankalpa (Intention), savasana atmosphere, or final journaling invitation.

COMPANION MATERIALS

THE ELEMENTAL TEACHING SPREAD

A spread for selecting class themes based on earth, water, fire, and air. Together, these four elements create a living cycle: Air clarifies, earth stabilizes, fire activates, and water replenishes — a balanced rhythm that mirrors both the tarot and the practices of yoga, breathwork, and meditation

Layout (four cards)

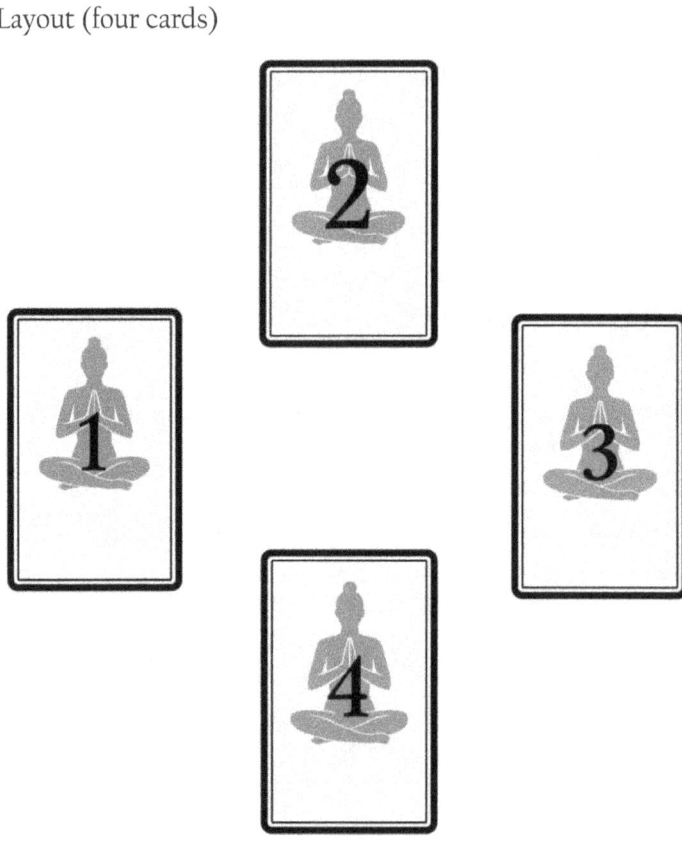

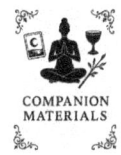

Imagine yourself in the center of these four cards. This layout mirrors the elemental cycle of earth, air, water, and fire around the practitioner.

Card 1 — Earth: What needs grounding?
This card reveals the physical or emotional foundation of the class.

Use it for:
- grounding asanas
- pacing
- the stability theme of the day

Card 2 — Water: What needs to flow or soften?
This card highlights emotional or intuitive elements.

Use it to guide:
- fluid sequencing
- vulnerability or emotional themes
- hips, pelvis, sacral focus
-

Card 3 — Fire: What needs to activate?
This card identifies energetic ignition or courage.

Use it to choose:
- your heat-building section
- core or strength work
- breath of fire or intentional intensity

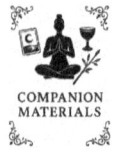

Card 4 — Air: What needs clarity?
This card guides mental spaciousness and insight.

Use it for:
- dharma language
- pranayama
- mindful pacing
- Sankalpa (Intention)s

This spread is excellent for classes themed around chakras, elemental cycles, or seasonal transitions.

COMPANION MATERIALS

THE TEACHER'S INSIGHT SPREAD

A deeper, introspective spread for teachers to guide their personal presence, voice, and alignment **before** holding space in class.

Layout (five cards)

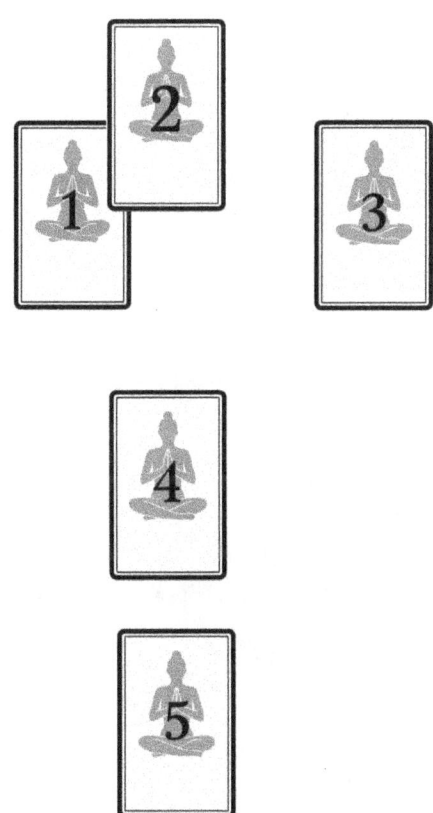

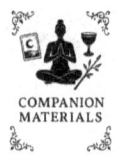

Card 1 — My Current Energy

What am I bringing into the room today?
This card helps you check in with yourself before getting on your mat.

Card 2 — How to Support My Students

What do my students need from me?
Guides tone, touch, cueing, music, breath choice.

Card 3 — How to Support Myself

What will help me hold space sustainably?
Guides self-care, boundaries, acuity with pacing or exertion.

Card 4 — The Lesson Beneath the Lesson

What subtle or spiritual theme is wanting to emerge?
Often aligns with the card that wants to be woven through the Dharma Talk.

Card 5 — Closing Heart Message

A blessing or takeaway for the class.
This becomes the Sankalpa (Intention), affirmation, or reflection.

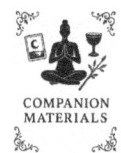

FIVE YAMAS TAROT SPREAD — "Living in Alignment"
A five-card spread that mirrors the energetic movement of the Yamas:
soften → clarify → balance → focus → release.

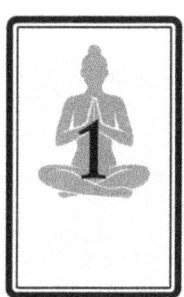 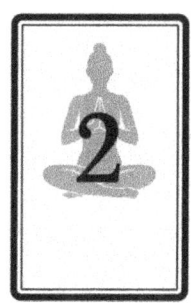 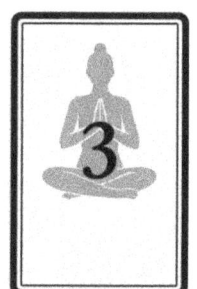

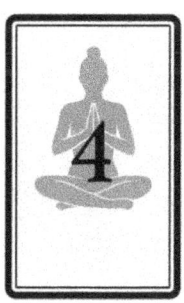 

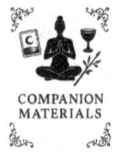

Card 1 — Ahiṁsa (Non-Harming / Compassion)

Where am I being called to soften, show compassion, or reduce harm — to myself or others?

Focus Points:

- Where harshness or pressure has built up
- What needs gentleness
- What requires healing presence

Card 2 — Satya (Truthfulness)

What truth do I need to acknowledge, speak, or align with right now?

Focus Points:

- Hidden truths
- Self-honesty
- Where clarity must replace illusion

Card 3 — Asteya (Non-Stealing / Generosity of Spirit)

Where am I holding back, taking too much, or undervaluing my own worth? Where can I practice generosity?

Focus Points:

- Energy leaks
- Scarcity mindset
- Unequal exchanges
- Opportunities to trust abundance

Card 4 — Brahmacharya (Right Use of Energy)

How can I direct my energy more intentionally toward what truly matters?

Focus Points:

- Recalibration
- Passion vs. depletion
- Boundaries
- Sacred focus + devotion

Card 5 — Aparigraha (Non-Attachment / Letting Go)

What am I being invited to release so I can move forward freely and lightly?

Focus Points:

- Clinging
- Old stories
- Past relationships or roles
- Attachments draining your prana

FIVE NIYAMAS TAROT SPREAD — "The Inner Path"
A five-card spread arranged in a gentle upward curve, reflecting the rise of consciousness through personal discipline and devotion.

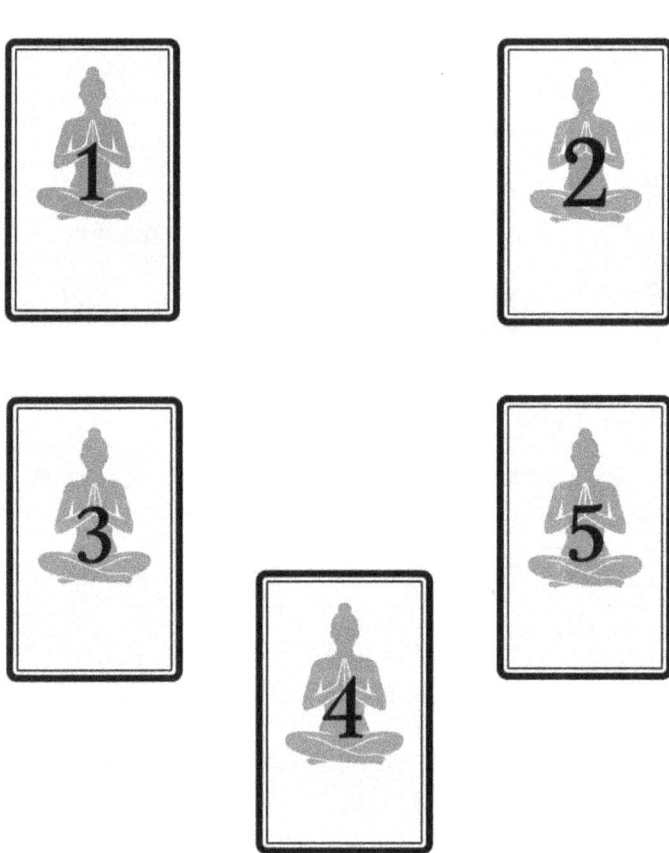

Card 1 — Sauca (Purification / Clarity)

What needs cleansing, clearing, or decluttering in my life, heart, or practice?

Focus Points:

- Energetic residue
- Emotional purification
- What needs to be rinsed away
- Space that wants to be opened

Card 2 — Santoṣa (Contentment / Peacefulness)

Where can I cultivate more contentment, gratitude, or acceptance in this moment?

Focus Points:

- What is already enough
- Where joy is available
- What can be softened into
- Present-moment peace

Card 3 — Tapas (Discipline / Inner Fire)

What practice, commitment, or effort is asking for my attention and consistent devotion?

Focus Points:

- Discipline without rigidity
- Where to apply heat
- Courage to continue
- Intentional effort

Card 4 — Svadhyaya (Self-Study / Inner Inquiry)

What do I need to learn about myself at this stage of my path? What truth is ready to be illuminated?

Focus Points:

- Inner patterns
- Sacred study
- Lessons emerging
- Wisdom wanting reflection

Card 5 — Isvara Praṇidhana (Surrender / Devotion)

What am I being called to surrender to the Divine, release control over, or trust more deeply?

Focus Points:

- Softening ego
- Trust in timing
- Devoting the practice
- Allowing grace to lead

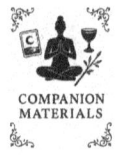

COMPANION MATERIALS

EIGHT-LIMBS OF YOGA TAROT SPREAD — "The Path of Integration"

This spread is arranged as a rising ladder or chakra-like column, reflecting the progression from outer discipline to inner awakening. See the glossary for more information these about the Eight Limbs.

(You can also lay it vertically if that feels more intuitive.)

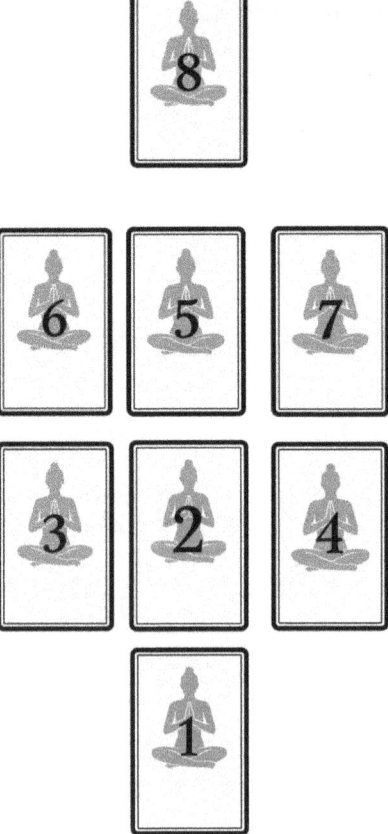

Card 1 — Yama (Ethical Restraints)

What ethical foundation or relational boundary needs attention in my life right now?

Focus Points:

- Integrity
- Non-harming
- Truth
- External alignment

Card 2 — Niyama (Personal Observances)

What personal practice, discipline, or inner state wants nurturing?

Focus Points:

- Purification
- Contentment
- Self-study
- Devotion

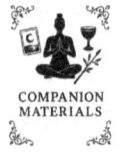

Card 3 — Asana (Embodiment)

What is my body communicating that needs to be honored, strengthened, or softened?

Focus Points:

- Somatic wisdom
- Grounding
- Strength vs. ease
- Physical truth

Card 4 — Praṇayama (Breath / Life-Force Regulation)

How can I work with breath or energy to expand my capacity and inner vitality?

Focus Points:

- Prana flow
- Where energy is stagnant
- What needs to be enlivened
- Breath rituals

Card 5 — Pratyahara (Withdrawal from External Pull)

What distractions or external influences am I ready to step back from?

Focus Points:

- Detachment from noise
- Turning inward
- Quieting sensory overload
- Energetic boundaries

Card 6 — Dharana (Concentration)

Where should I direct my focused attention? What requires single-pointed clarity?

Focus Points:

- Mental discipline
- Choosing one priority
- Avoiding diffusion
- Intentionality

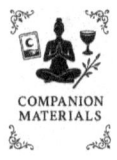

Card 7 — Dhyana (Meditation)

What practice or mindset will help me settle into sustained presence and awareness?

Focus Points:

- Stillness
- Flow state
- Presence
- Non-judgmental awareness

Card 8 — Samadhi (Unity / Bliss)

What higher wisdom, integration, or spiritual truth is ready to emerge?

Focus Points:

- Transcendence
- Wholeness
- Union
- Liberation
- Grace

COMPANION MATERIALS

CLASS SHEET

A structured guide for intentional, tarot-informed yoga. This template can be used for journaling or planning your class or practice.

CLASS TITLE:

DATE / TIME:

TAROT CARD OR SPREAD USED:
(Write the card(s) drawn, or the spread used.)

PRIMARY THEME:
(One sentence expressing the core message of the class.)

SUPPORTING THEMES:
(Emotional, energetic, philosophical, archetypal.)

CLASS/PRACTICE SEQUENCE

1. DHARMA TALK (Opening 2-3 minutes)

Key message: _____

Supporting imagery / symbols: _____

Archetype connection (Major Arcana, Cups, Wands, Swords, Pentacles): _____

Notes:

_____

_____

_____

_____

_____

_____

_____

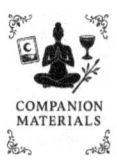

2. BREATHWORK (Pranayama)

Choose one:
- ☐ Nadi Shodhana
- ☐ Ujjayi
- ☐ Sama Vritti
- ☐ Kapalabhati
- ☐ Box Breath
- ☐ Other: _____

Cues to emphasize:

_____

_____

_____

3. MUDRA SELECTION

- ☐ Anjali
- ☐ Gyan / Jnana
- ☐ Varuna
- ☐ Hridaya
- ☐ Agni
- ☐ Other: _____

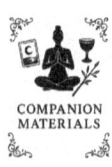

Why this mudra for today's theme?

_____

_____

4. WARM-UP (Opening Movement)

Opening shapes:

_____

_____

_____

Joint mobilization / gentle flow:

_____

_____

_____

Key Cues:

_____

_____

_____

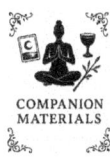

Notes:

_____

_____

_____

5. MAIN SEQUENCE

(peak pose, energetic arc, transitions)

Peak Pose / Central Shape:

_____

Supporting Postures:

1. _____
2. _____
3. _____
4. _____
5. _____

Energetic Focus:

☐ Grounding
☐ Flowing
☐ Heat-building
☐ Expansion
☐ Balance
☐ Restoration

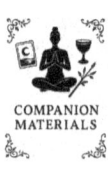

Key sequencing notes:

_____

_____

_____

6. COOL-DOWN & INTEGRATION

Stretching or softening shapes:

_____

_____

_____

Breath Cues:

_____

_____

_____

Emotional/energetic unwinding:

_____

_____

_____

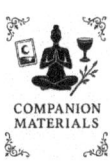

Notes:

_____

_____

_____

_____

_____

7. SANKALPA (INTENTION) (2–3 minutes)

Guiding message:

_____

_____

Affirmation or mantra:

_____

_____

8. FINAL NOTES FOR NEXT TIME

What landed? What to refine? What students needed?

_____

_____

_____

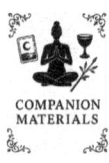

9. MY PERSONAL TAKEAWAY

COMPANION MATERIALS

USING THIS GUIDE FOR YOUR PRACTICE

This section offers a simple, step-by-step walkthrough of how to bring *Asana & Arcana* into your personal practice or teaching. While the book is rich with symbolism, sequencing, and contemplative material, it is designed to be used intuitively — a companion you can return to whenever you need inspiration, clarity, or an energetic theme for your movement or meditation. This demonstration shows how to move from drawing a Tarot card to creating a meaningful, embodied experience on the mat. Whether you are a teacher planning a class or a student cultivating a home practice, this guide helps you understand how each element of the book fits together in a practical and nourishing way.

At its heart, this demonstration highlights the relationship between reflection and embodiment. Tarot offers the symbolic lens through which we explore our inner landscape, while yoga gives us the physical and energetic tools to move that insight through the body. By following the steps in these pages, you will learn how to translate a card's message into breathwork, movement, contemplation, and meditation — creating a practice that feels cohesive, intuitive, and deeply personal. Think of this as your orientation into a new way of practicing: one that honors the wisdom of the cards and the intelligence of the body in equal measure.

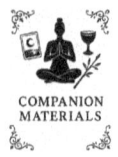

COMPANION MATERIALS

1. Begin by Drawing a Card

Start your practice by selecting one tarot card — either intuitively, randomly, or deliberately. Take a moment to look at the imagery, notice what feelings arise, and read the card's main theme in the corresponding section of this book. This becomes the anchor for your practice: the emotional, energetic, or symbolic quality that will guide your movement and breath.

For our demonstration, I drew the Knight of Cups. Referring back to the Realm of Cups section in the book and finding the Knight, we can see that this card represents heart-led action; the theme of the class being romanticism, inspiration, and moving from feeling.

2. Read the Dharma Talk and Reflection

Turn to the dharma talk for that card and read it slowly, allowing the message to settle in the body. Let the language help you understand the core teaching: Is this a moment for grounding? Expansion? Clarity? Softening? Insight? Whether you're teaching or practicing independently, the dharma talk sets the tone and intention of the practice.

The Knight of Cup symbolizes following the heart's calling - following this, my opening Dharma Talk would be:

As you breathe here, notice what it feels like to release the need to perform, to impress, or to strive. Let the breath move in and out of the body like a gentle tide, clearing space around the heart. With every inhale, feel into the truth of what you want — not what you think you should want, not what others expect, but what quietly stirs beneath the

surface. With every exhale, imagine letting go of the ego's agenda: the pressure to perfect, to push, to prove.

As you settle into practice today, ask yourself:
Where is my heart leading me?
Not the mind, not the habit, not the fear — the heart. The soft, steady compass that always knows when something is for you and when it is not. Let this question sit gently in your chest as you breathe, as you move, as you open into the shapes ahead.

Take in one more long inhale, allowing a dream, a desire, or a truth to rise to the surface.
Take a slow, releasing exhale, letting it be enough simply to feel it.

Your practice today is not about effort. It is about sincerity.
Let the heart lead — the body will follow.

3. Explore the Suggested Breathwork (Pranayama)

Each card includes breathwork practices chosen for their energetic resonance. Pause and notice how the recommended pranayama supports the theme of the card. For grounding cards, breath may be slow and steady; for energizing cards, it may be warming or activating; for emotional cards, it may focus on spaciousness or release. Take a few rounds to feel the shift they create.

Nadi Shodhana, the pranayama associated with the Realm of Cups, helps to balance the emotional state. After the opening meditation and Dharma talk, sit comfortably supporting your right elbow in your left pal. Press your right thumb against your right nostril to close it;

COMPANION MATERIALS

inhaling through your left nostril. Release your thumb. Then press your right ring finger against your left nostril to close it, exhaling through your left nostril. Continue inhaling through the right nostril and exhaling through the left, taking slow, relaxed breaths and thinking moving your breath through your heart.

4. Move Into the Asana and Mudra Suggestions

Refer to the asanas and mudras associated with that particular card, guided by the section introduction for the suit or arcana. These postures are not meant to be followed rigidly but to inspire the energetic direction of your practice. Use the poses as a framework: whether you're teaching a full sequence or practicing a few intuitive shapes, let the card's theme guide your choices.

The asanas for the Realm of Cups include cat-caw, seated forward fold, low lunge, and reclined bound angle. Suggested mudras are Varuna mudra and Hridaya mudra – both supporting emotional flow, openness and compassion. Be willing to move with honesty; stepping into a pose with knowing and leaving ego behind. Shape the pose to meet your body where it is today; don't try to shape your body to fit the pose.

Sit comfortably after completing several rounds of Nadi Shodhana, let's open our practice with Hridaya mudra. Curl your index finger in touching the base of your thumb; bring the tips of your middle and ring fingers to the tip of your thumb; your little finger remains straight. Turn your attention to the feeling of connection between your thumb and fingers. This gesture supports emotional openness and compassion

for your practice today. Breathe in these words: I move from the wisdom of my heart.

5. Shape Your Sequence or Personal Flow

Using the card's theme, the breathwork, and the suggested postures, weave together a mini-practice or full class. The key is cohesion: each element should echo the heart of the card. For example, grounding cards may call for slow, steady movement and long holds; heart-centered cards may invite softness and fluidity; fire cards may inspire strength and activation. Let intuition and embodiment shape the sequence.

After warming up, start on hands and knees with cat-cow. Allow yourself to move in any way that feels good. Think about opening and lifting your heart with each inhalation.

From here, swing your legs forward and take a seat. Reach your arms high, adding a little tension between your shoulder blades to open your chest. Inhale deeply to expand your heart space as you reach forward with your chest and hinge at the hips. Show yourself compassion by going only as far as you safely can. Use blocks under your forehead for support, if you want. Relax here simply enjoying the length of your spine. Gently use your hands to press your body upright, letting your head come up last. Take a few breaths here mindfully coming upright.

Come to standing. Step forward with your right foot, bending your knee. Gently lower your left knee to the ground. Here consider padding your knee with a blanket for comfort. Get your balance. On a deep inhale, reach your arms to the sky; on the next exhale, settle into your

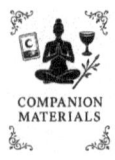

hips, deepening the pose. Think about how you're feeling. Can you find some ease with this effort? Where can you soften? Do you want to reach higher and possibly offer your heart to the sky in a soft backbend?

After repeating your low lunge on the other side and including any other asanas that your body wants today, lie down on your back, padding your head with a blanket. Touch the soles of your feet together and let your knees open to the sides. Note how you feel. Do you want support? If so, ease blocks under your thigh bones. Open your heart to whatever you may receive. Relax into the mat.

6. Close With the Card's Meditation

End your practice by reading or offering the sankalpa or a closing meditation of your choice. Use these words to help integrate the card's message into the body, breath, and mind. Take a few moments to sit with the sensations and insights that have emerged, trusting that the practice has helped reveal exactly what needed attention.

Let's close this practice with the varuna mudra. Touch the tip of your little finger to the tip of your finger, letting your other fingers reman straight and relaxed. Turn your attention to the contact points and where you can feel the warmth of your fingers touching your thumb. Breathe in these words: I move from the wisdom of my heart.

7. Optional: Journal or Reflect

If you'd like to deepen the experience, turn to the journaling prompts or simply reflect on how the card's energy showed up in your body. Teachers may choose to record what themes resonated, which movements supported the message, and how the card might inform future classes.

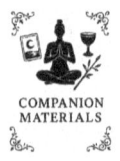

Let's work through the class/practice planning worksheet together:

CLASS TITLE: *Wisdom of the Heart*

DATE / TIME: *Monday, 7pm hatha class*

TAROT CARD OR SPREAD USED:
(Write the card(s) drawn, or the spread used.)

Knight of Cups

PRIMARY THEME:
(One sentence expressing the core message of the class.)

Listen to your heart and move with intention

SUPPORTING THEMES:
(Emotional, energetic, philosophical, archetypal.)

Allow yourself to open and receive; find support where you want it; be open to allowing yourself the freedom of movement

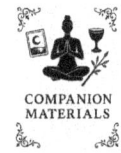

COMPANION MATERIALS

CLASS/PRACTICE SEQUENCE

1. DHARMA TALK (Opening 2–3 minutes)

Key message:

Release the need to impress; remove expectations – your own and those of others

Supporting imagery / symbols:

Gentle tide of the breath; allowing your heart to lead; to be a compass

Archetype connection (Major Arcana, Cups, Wands, Swords, Pentacles):

The Realm of Cups

Notes:

Allow seven minutes for the opening meditation and dharma talk

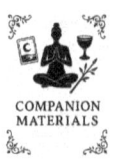

2. BREATHWORK (Pranayama)

Choose one:
- ✓ Nadi Shodhana
- ☐ Ujjayi
- ☐ Sama Vritti
- ☐ Kapalabhati
- ☐ Box Breath
- ☐ Other: _____

Cues to emphasize:

Stay relaxed; focus on deep, slow, easy breaths

3. MUDRA SELECTION

- ☐ Anjali
- ☐ Gyan / Jnana
- ✓ Varuna
- ✓ Hridaya
- ☐ Agni
- ☐ Other: _____

Why this mudra for today's theme?

Both mudras allow for compassion and fluidity

4. WARM-UP (Opening Movement)

Opening shapes:

Seated meditation; supported fish pose; shoulder rolls

Joint mobilization / gentle flow:

Cat-cow with student-led variations

Key Cues:

"Allow yourself to move as you want." "How do you feel in this pose?" "Can you find ease? Soften? Show yourself compassion?"

Notes:

Encourage students to close their eyes if they have a hard time moving without watching others.

5. MAIN SEQUENCE

(peak pose, energetic arc, transitions)

Peak Pose / Central Shape:

Low lunge with slight backbend

Supporting Postures:

Standing stretch – option for soft backbend
Chair (to warm up thighs)
High lunge

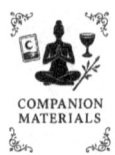
COMPANION MATERIALS

Energetic Focus:

✓ Grounding
✓ Flowing
☐ Heat-building
✓ Expansion
☐ Balance
☐ Restoration

Key sequencing notes:

Slow, fluid-like movements; connect breath to movement; remind students to open their hearts and take time to do what feels right in their bodies

6. COOL-DOWN & INTEGRATION

Stretching or softening shapes:

Seated forward fold; reclined bound angle

Breath Cues:

Soften; deepen, breath deeply into your chest/heart space

Emotional/energetic unwinding:

Close with Hridaya mudra

7. SANKALPA (INTENTION) (2–3 minutes)

Guiding message:

Listen to your body; honor what it's telling you; relax into its purpose for this class

Affirmation or mantra:

I move from the wisdom of my heart

8. FINAL NOTES FOR NEXT TIME

What landed? What to refine? What students needed?

Remove standing poses; remain closer to the ground; students appreciated the longer period in final relaxation and taking the time to come back to themselves before class ended.

9. MY PERSONAL TAKEAWAY:

A very relaxing class! Some found it difficult to move with little or no guidance. Think about adding trusting yourself when teaching the next time.

As you can see, this demonstration shows how each part of the book works together to help you create a meaningful, intuitive, and embodied practice. With experience, the process becomes fluid — a seamless blend of reflection, movement, and inner listening.

CLOSING BLESSING

May the wisdom you cultivated here continue to move within you.
As breath settles and the body softens, may clarity rise gently to the surface.
May what you discovered—through stillness, through movement, through feeling—
take root in your heart with steadiness and grace.

May the archetypes you touched today walk beside you,
not as forces outside you,
but as reflections of your own resilience, intuition, courage, and tenderness.

May you move forward with a grounded spine,
an open heart,
and a mind spacious enough to hold both mystery and truth.

May your steps be guided by presence,
your choices shaped by compassion,
and your life illuminated by the quiet brilliance that already lives within you.

May you walk down a path of light and love and happiness.

Go gently.
Go bravely.
Go blessed.

GLOSSARY

Anjali Mudra
A gesture of reverence made by pressing the palms together at the heart center; symbolizes unity, gratitude, and inner balance.

Arcana
A term referring to the two sections of the tarot: the Major Arcana (archetypal experiences) and the Minor Arcana (everyday themes).

Asana
Physical postures practiced in yoga to cultivate strength, stability, mobility, and mindful awareness.

Breathwork (see Pranayama)
The intentional regulation of the breath to support physical, emotional, and energetic balance.

Chakras
Subtle energy centers within the body that influence emotional, physical, and spiritual well-being. The seven main Chakras are:

- **Root Chakra (Muladhara):** Located at the base of the spine, it's associated with survival, security, and grounding.
- **Sacral Chakra (Svadhisthana):** Situated in the lower abdomen, it governs emotions, creativity, and sensuality.

- **Solar Plexus Chakra (Manipura):** Found in the upper abdomen, it's linked to personal power, confidence, and willpower.
- **Heart Chakra (Anahata):** Located at the center of the chest, it is the bridge between the lower and upper chakras and is associated with love, compassion, and emotional healing.
- **Throat Chakra (Vishuddha):** Found in the throat area, it governs communication, self-expression, and truth.
- **Third Eye Chakra (Ajna):** Located between the eyebrows, it is connected to intuition, insight, and wisdom.
- **Crown Chakra (Sahasrara):** Positioned at the top of the head, it represents spiritual connection, consciousness, and enlightenment.

Dharana
Concentration; the sixth limb of yoga, focused on holding attention on a single point.

Dharma Talk
A short teaching or reflection offered at the beginning of a yoga class to set intention and guide inner awareness.

Dhyana
Meditation; the seventh limb of yoga, describing sustained, effortless awareness.

Eight Limbs of Yoga
A complete framework from the *Yoga Sutra* describing ethical principles, physical practice, breath regulation, concentration, meditation, and spiritual integration.

Gyan Mudra
A hand gesture touching the thumb and index finger; used to enhance focus, clarity, and intuitive awareness.

Hatha Yoga
Hatha yoga is a foundational branch of yoga that generally includes asana (poses), pranayama (breathwork), and meditation. It's generally a slower-paced style of yoga with several breaths spent in each pose.

Inversions
An inversion in yoga is any asana (pose) where the head is below the heart. It can be a forward fold, a backbend, or a headstand, among others.

Major Arcana
The 22 archetypal cards of the tarot that represent universal life lessons, spiritual evolution, and transformative experiences.

Meditation
A practice of stillness and awareness used to quiet the mind, regulate the nervous system, and deepen inner connection.

Minor Arcana
The 56 cards of the tarot divided into four suits—Cups, Wands, Swords, and Pentacles—representing everyday experiences, emotions, thoughts, and actions.

Mudra
A symbolic hand gesture or energetic seal used in yoga and meditation to direct attention and shape inner experience.

Pranayama
Breath regulation practices designed to expand, steady, or refine life force energy (*prana*).

Pratyahara
Withdrawal from the senses; the fifth limb of yoga, redirecting awareness inward by reducing external distraction.

Samadhi
A state of integration and unity; the eighth limb of yoga, described as peaceful, embodied awareness and connection.

Sequencing
The intentional arrangement of yoga postures to support physical safety, energetic flow, and thematic clarity.

Tarot
A symbolic system of 78 cards used for introspection, reflection, and understanding universal and personal archetypes.

Theme
The central idea or energetic focus guiding a yoga class; in this book, each class theme aligns with one tarot card.

Vinyasa Yoga
Vinyasa yoga is a foundational branch of yoga that generally includes asana (poses), pranayama (breathwork), and meditation. It's a faster-paced style of yoga moving through asanas at the pace of your breath – linking movement with breath.

Yama
Ethical guidelines related to how we interact with the world; the first limb of yoga.

Yoga
A holistic system of physical, mental, energetic, and spiritual practices that cultivate presence, awareness, and union.

Yoga Nidra
A meditative, guided practice of conscious rest that induces profound relaxation and inner awareness.

Yogi / Yogini
A practitioner of yoga.

Thank you for spending time with *Asana & Arcana*. As a gesture of gratitude, I invite you to download this complimentary companion ebook, **A Gift of Practice: Tarot Reflections to Support Your Yoga Journey**. Inside, you'll find simple, grounding tarot spreads designed to support reflection, embodiment, and presence—on the mat and in everyday life. May this offering meet you gently and deepen your practice in quiet, meaningful ways.

To download your free copy, simply click on the link below or scan the QR code.

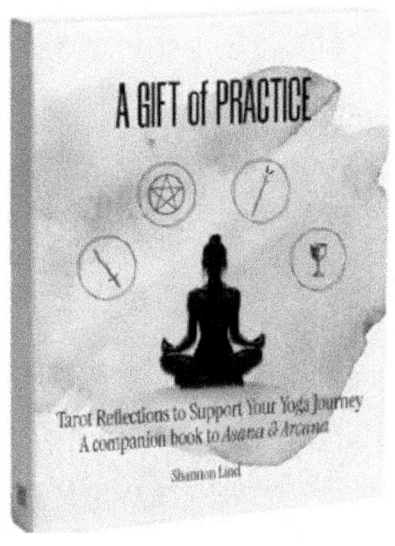

Continue your practice with **A Gift of Practice**, *a free tarot companion for yoga practitioners and teachers*
https://shannonlindyoga.kit.com/2dd452004e

www.ingramcontent.com/pod-product-compliance
Lightning Source LLC
Chambersburg PA
CBHW070626030426
42337CB00020B/3929